Hot Point Fitness

DEDICATION

I would like to dedicate this book to the three most influential people in my life: my father, Dr. Abraham Zimelman, my wife Jodi, and the memory of my mother, Cookie.

SPECIAL THANKS

I would like to give thanks to the following people for their support and encouragement. Thanks to Vince Scully, the legendary voice of the Los Angeles Dodgers, for noticing. My deepest thanks to David Brokaw for loving baseball and introducing me to the greatest agent, Mel Berger. Thanks to the good people of Perseus, most especially Marnie Cochran for shepherding this book through all phases and always lending a hand, Lissa Warren for the great pub, and Marco Pavia for putting on the finishing touches in time. Thanks to Doulas Cloutier for the wonderful photographs. My gratitude to Bob Hughes, Bill Hughes, Bobby Hughes, Big Show, Aaron Boone, Ryan Stromsborg, Gabe Alvarez, Chad Moeller, Jeff Cirillo, Larry Schrier and Doug Williams, your hard work is a living testament to this program. Thanks also to Dennis Weiss, Stanford Tabb, Evi Dresser, Debbie Goldfarb, Irv and Shirley Rubenstein, Dr. Alice Zimelman, Mark Bell, Cohen Duncan, Salter Giddens, Vance McDaniel, Adam Strand, Jon Williams, Latoya Odom, J.J. Cohen, and Milena Castiel, and an especially warm set of thanks to Ilana and Eric Zimelman. Mark Laska, thank you for making my vision speak. Carli, Taylor, and Humphrey . . . one day you'll be able to read this too. Dad loves you.

HOT POINT FITNESS

The Revolutionary New Program for Fast and Total Body Transformation

STEVE ZIM
MARK LASKA

PERSEUS PUBLISHING
Cambridge, Massachusetts

Library of Congress Control Number: 2002102005
ISBN 0-7382-0603-2

Perseus Publishing is a member of the Perseus Books Group.

Find us on the World Wide Web at http://www.perseuspublishing.com

Perseus Publishing books are available at special discounts for bulk purchases in the U.S. by corporations, insti-tutions, and other organizations. For more information, please contact the Special Markets Department at the Perseus Books Group, 11 Cambridge Center, Cambridge, MA, 02142, or call 1-617-252-5298.

Text design by Jeff Williams
Set in 11-point Slimbach by the Perseus Books Group

First paperback printing, March 2002
1 2 3 4 5 6 7 8 9 10—04 03 02

Contents

Introduction

I own and operate a fitness center in Los Angeles. The facility is manned by a small army of personal trainers. Each of these trainers teaches the Hot Point Fitness program to our clients. The clientele who come to this facility work with a devoted personal trainer on a one-on-one basis. Over the years I have personally witnessed the transformation of literally thousands of people that have subscribed to the Hot Point method. These people have come in all forms, shapes, sizes, and ages. Hot Point is effective for everyone that gives it their all. While I have personally trained elderly, disabled, and extremely obese people and helped them to achieve a level of fitness and wellness that they did not think was possible, the majority of my clients are celebrities and professional athletes.

For celebrities and athletes, the highest degree of physical appearance and optimum physical performance are not only highly desirable but also a necessity to earn a living. Their paychecks are drawn not on the premise of *if* they can get into shape but rather on the degree of their physical fitness. While these particular people come to me in relatively good condition, it is their desire to further improve their appearance and performance. Most of the athletes that I train are not football players, wrestlers, or Olympic weight lifters—athletes that depend on sheer bulk. The majority of athletes that I train depend on physical strength, agility, flexibility, and speed to be successful in their sport. Over the years I have developed a reputation among Olympic figure skaters and professional baseball players for being able to help them increase their performance levels.

I tend to think of figure skaters and baseball players as prototypical athletic bodies. I mention these two body types only to point out that Hot Point Fitness is the perfect program for the average person, and that it is not my hidden agenda to reconfigure your body into that of the Incredible Hulk. Neither skaters nor baseball players must be tremendously tall or massively muscular to excel. In fact, such physical attributes may impede their athleticism. When we stand next to them, we say to ourselves, "Yeah, that could be me. I could do that if I had the skills." With Hot Point Fitness, you can undoubtedly work your way towards that level of fitness. In fact, you may be using the very same program your favorite actor or athlete is using to get in and stay in shape.

What truly separates you or me from the professional athlete is not how we train but the reason *why* we train. This brings me to an interesting point. How would you train if you were training for the Olympics? How would you train if you were training to run in a marathon? How would you train if you were going to be in a bodybuilding competition? Because we live in a goal-oriented society, I feel that it is an interesting question to address. Would we train differently if we were training for an event?

One of my favorite clients posed this theory to me the other day. He said, "If I sold my business tomorrow and I didn't have to work, and had all this time on my hands, what would I do?" He pondered for a moment and said, "I think I would come in and hire you to train me to be a professional bodybuilder." This client is over 50, is not especially muscular, and looks nothing like what you would picture when you think of a bodybuilder. He replied, "If I could build myself up to that level, what would it take?" Only then did it dawn on me that he was actually quite serious. He was contemplating selling his business and was concerned with what he would do with his free time. He then confirmed my suspicion. "If I could train myself for a bodybuilding show," he added, "how could that possibly hurt me? I would get in fantastic condition and do what I am doing now just to maintain what I had achieved." He then asked me one final question. "What would it take for me, what would I have to do exactly, so I could reach my goal?"

My client, brilliant man that he is, had struck upon something. If we are absolutely driven to reach our goals, why do we insist upon mediocrity when we set those goals? If instead of "losing five pounds," we set our sights on running a marathon, or training for a bodybuilding contest, where would we end up? If you could train at the level of a professional athlete, what level of condition would you be in a month from now? If you could sustain that level of exercise for two months, what would you look like? What if you could do that for six months or a year? As I explained everything he would need to do to train for such an event, it made a great deal of sense to provide the exact same information to you.

This inspired me to create a plan for everyone who reads this book. No matter where you are in the transformational process, whatever fitness level you currently enjoy, no matter what age or physical ability, you can take yourself to the level that you desire. This book represents a game plan to take the person who is a couch potato to the fitness level of a professional athlete. If you have led a sedentary life or have not exercised in years, or, like my insightful client, you were in relatively good shape but wanted to be in the ultimate shape, there are a few steps to reach this heightened level of fitness.

Think of this book as if it were an owner's manual for your body. In this book you will find all the information that you will need to reach whatever fitness level you desire... and beyond. The book will discuss the three ingredients of your transformation, and then walk you through the process of your transformation step by step. I have written this book to simulate the experience of having your own personal trainer. And for each day you are to work out, I have planned exactly what you should do to achieve your goal. I have spent the better part of my life perfecting and fine-tuning this program. It is my life and my life's work that I share with you.

PART 1

The Hot Point Fitness Way

A Positive Addiction

Working <u>With</u> Your Body's Innate Desires

The point is to become an addict. Not an addict to drugs, alcohol, sex, or gambling, but to form an addiction to something that empowers you . . . an addiction that makes you feel great about yourself . . . an addiction that enables you to look and feel your best . . . an addiction that will add years and quality to your life . . . an addiction to doing something positive, feeling positive, and projecting that positivity into everything that you do and to everyone who you come in contact with.

Unless you have been living on a remote island without satellite TV, we have all been victimized by empty promises. All of us are constantly bombarded by products that promise to make us slimmer, to make us more beautiful, to make us healthier, to help us be more productive, to be more attractive, or promise to answer our prayers and to finally and forever make us happy at last. Every time we open a newspaper, stand in the checkout line at the grocery store, or turn on the television, we are in essence being told that we are not good enough as we are—that we need to be slimmer to be more appealing, that we need to be better, or faster, or stronger, or healthier, or younger, or more beautiful people than we are now. Advertisers prey upon our vanity. Being younger, slimmer, and healthier is in one way or another attached to a product. This bottled supplement, diet, article, or exercise gizmo is something that we absolutely must buy at this very moment or we will surely perish a horrible death. The promise of a new and improved you compels us to order from the infomercial, to buy the book or magazine, or to rent a moving van and crew of five to bring home the piece of equipment that will finally get our thighs slender. More often than not, the equipment (which is just slightly smaller than an elephant) ends up being a very expensive clothes rack. You eventually become frustrated and quite possibly offensive to those around you by living on a subsistence of grapefruit and onions . . . and the last time you saw that article on getting the perfect buns was when you de-crumbed the toaster and threw the whole lot into the recycling bin. The more products we see that promise a "new you," the more disgusted we get with the whole notion of changing. We become sick and tired of the magic pill promising to make us 50 pounds lighter and increase our IQ by 300 points in *just one week*. We become suspicious and cynical when we are forced to think about changing. We all are sickened by empty promises. I promise not to make you an empty promise. My only promise to you is that there is no hidden potion, no magic pill, no miracle, no fairy-tale solution that will enable you to get slimmer, fit, or healthy, other than putting the time and effort it takes into achieving these life-changing qualities.

But, I want to assure you that you can indeed change your life for the better. You can become slimmer and leaner. You can create muscle tone. You can become healthier and live a longer and more active life. You can indeed create more bone density and offset the aging process. You can improve the strength and resilience of your heart. Change is possible . . . even probable. However, this change will not occur over night. Change cannot possibly happen as quickly as we would like. This change will happen in small increments over time. The length of time to actually see these dramatic changes will vary for each individual, but if you can commit yourself, this change will undoubtedly, without exception, occur for you.

I am certain that you just want to tear into this book and get started, but just a few words before you begin. There are some important considerations that should be taken into account. We all come in different shapes and sizes, and all with our own individual needs. I cannot possibly guess what your goals are, so you must take some mental notes for yourself. Whatever got you started, whatever motivated you to buy this book, or pushed you to seriously consider exercising, is a very important thing to note for yourself. It is, in fact, a key to motivate you towards an end result. You may have been motivated to buy this book so that you could shed some unwanted pounds or to create better muscle tone. Some are searching for a way to improve their overall health. These are great motivating factors, and it is important to remind yourself of them frequently for some time to come. However, because change happens more slowly than we might like, these motivating factors may not be enough, in and of themselves, to make you incorporate an exercise and nutrition strategy for the long haul.

And the long haul is indeed the goal. This is not just a system to take you from point A to point Z, but to help you at every point in between, and also be a program to use throughout your entire lifetime. You will find that after just a few short weeks you will be feeling much differently than you do today. You will notice you have more energy. You will notice that you don't "crash" in the afternoon hours. You may feel more vital than you have felt in years, or maybe even in your entire life. You might finally get a full night's sleep, and feel fully rested when you wake up in the morning. You will find that you can handle stress more easily. You will not be edgy, or irritable, or easily aggravated. You will notice a sense of clarity in your thought process. You may become more productive at work, you may find yourself brainstorming creative ideas, or able to perceive the subliminal subtlety of a situation. You may notice that your skin looks better and that your hair is thicker and healthier. You may carry around a euphoric feeling of giddiness. You may find yourself singing in the shower for the first time in a long time. You may acquire a bit of a swagger when you walk, develop an air of confidence, and finally come to believe that you really are as good as you think you are. You may find yourself actually feeling sexy, you may feel more amorous than you have ever felt, or you may discover that your sex drive is greatly enhanced and you are becoming a walking sexual dynamo. In short, you will have much more to look forward to than a new wardrobe.

Feeling all of these amazingly positive things on a daily basis is addictive. The point of this book is not to merely look better but to form a habit and to have that habit blossom into a full-blown addiction. Certainly you will look fantastic down the road, and that is your ultimate payoff, but you will be rewarded in thousands of ways each and every day, and that is precisely what is so addictive. This addiction is perhaps the only addiction that could in any way, shape, or form be construed as "positive." I guarantee that you will not need to check into the Betty Ford Center, enroll in a twelve-step program, or be in need of an intervention after you have declared yourself a Hot Point Junkie.

Forming a habit takes a certain and specific amount of time. Experts, scientists, and numerous twelve-step programs have determined that it takes approximately 21 days to break an old or "negative" habit, and conversely to form a new one. The Hot Point Program is designed in three phases specifically to enable you to form this habit. Each phase has a starting point and an ending point. Each phase will last for 28 days and gradually enables you to increase your stamina and strength in tangible increments. At the end of Phase One, you will have successfully incorporated and assimilated regular exercise into your life. By the end of Phase Two, you will find yourself needing to do it, and also feeling sluggish and not quite yourself if you don't. At the end of Phase Three, you will be as fit as you have ever been with more strength, flexibility, and endurance than you have ever enjoyed in your entire life.

To begin your personal journey of "positive addiction" all that is required is that you set aside one hour of your day, three times a week. Before we go any further, get out your organizer, consult the nearest calendar, or log onto your computerized scheduling device. Simply reserve an hour three times a week for the next two weeks. Without even thinking about it, get the calendar and find three days this week when you can squeeze in an hour. C'mon . . . Make the commitment . . . that's not too much to ask of yourself, is it? Think Nike: "Just do it!" Now schedule in week two. That was easy enough wasn't it? The ancient Chinese philosopher Lao-Tzu said, "The journey of a thousand miles begins with one step." Congratulate yourself, because you just made that first step. This is a journey that will greatly enrich and quite possibly lengthen your life.

You have made a commitment to try this program out for the next two weeks. Now it is time to hand over the reins. I have been a personal trainer for years and have taken so many people through a process of transformation that I have lost count. Essentially, I am training you to be your own personal trainer. Unfortunately for me, I will not be able to be at your side for your transformation. Fortunately for you, I have created this book to be exactly like the experience of having a personal trainer at your side. I have set up exercise programs for thousands of people and walked them through the entire process. Whether they are elderly, have health problems, are experiencing pain, or are in top physical condition, the program I have created is easy to follow. With this book, you have all the information you will need for your journey. With a little help, you are now going to be your own coach.

Think of this book as if it were an owner's manual. Instead of referring to a blender, a VCR, or a car, this owner's manual is primarily concerned with your body. By following the directions in this owner's manual you will have all the information needed to give you the highest performance possible, to keep you in the best condition, and to maintain that prime condition for the life of your investment. In this owner's manual you will find step-by-step directions to transform a junkyard heap into a showpiece, or to turn a showpiece into a highly valuable commodity. This owner's manual is not a generalized program that will be exactly the same for everyone. Although the Hot Point System is designed to take the body that is inactive to the fitness level of a professional athlete, there are many levels in between. Based upon your individual goals, or your intended end result, you will find a road map to your destination within these covers. Whether you exercise regularly, whether you have not been physically active for many years, whether you want to shed some pounds, or whether you want to gain muscle mass, you will discover that this program is designed to meet your individual needs.

The Hot Point Program is simple. The book does not espouse several theories, leaving you to decide which may be the best solution. Instead it has been created to simulate the experience you would have with your own personal trainer, meaning that it is a structured series of directions to take you to a final destination. Hot Point Fitness is solely dedicated to your personal transformation, and there will be many steps along that path. The path has three milestones, namely, Phase One, Phase Two, and Phase Three. This is not a race where your ultimate objective is to pass each milestone. The ultimate objective is to simply stay on the path. You may decide that the first phase of this program allows you to reach your goal. You may choose to stay at this level for the rest of your life. You may decide that the physical challenge of Phase Two or Phase Three is better suited for your needs . . . it doesn't really matter. Again, the only thing that matters is to stay on the path. For every day of exercise, a specific workout has been designed especially for you. All three phases have three common factors: aerobic activity, resistance or weight training, and nutritional guidelines. All you have to do is follow the directions.

You will find that by following the directions, you are being guided along the path of physical transformation. After just a week on this path, you will feel the difference. After two weeks, you will begin to see these changes in the mirror. After four weeks, others will notice and begin commenting. These changes are fantastic. They make us feel great about what we are doing for ourselves. They keep us on the path. Perhaps even more dramatic than these physical changes will be the way that you feel about yourself.

Not only is Hot Point Fitness designed to transform your body, but you will soon discover that the workout is designed to create a sense of accomplishment. When you are exercising, you will be performing a certain number of repetitions. When you have completed the prescribed number, you will have completed a set. With each repetition, you will be concentrating on performing an exercise to perfection. Each time you do this, it will be seen as a personal victory. For every set completed, you will have had many successive victories. By the time you have finished your workout for the day, you will have been a winner so many times that you create a pattern for yourself. As you will see, this pattern of success becomes addictive and will give you an earned sense of achievement. Carry this sense of achievement out of the gym and apply it to the rest of your daily activities—to your work, to your relationships, to everything that you do.

2

Mastering Your Body

The Mental Process Behind Your Physical Efforts

While the final destination of your journey is a physical transformation, the experience of achieving small victories on a daily basis will keep you on the path toward your ultimate goal. Most people who exercise regularly are doing so because of the way it makes them feel. Yes, it will make you feel good physically, but what will make you feel great is the way that you feel about yourself as a result of the physical accomplishment. There is a mind-set, a headspace, a mood-altering, a self-esteem shift that occurs when you exercise, and exercise regularly. Since it is precisely this mental aspect of the workout that is so life-changing, I would like to spend this chapter talking about how to get the greatest mental return on this investment in your physical fitness.

We give a lot of lip service to the concept of a mind/body connection. This term has become the hottest concept in exercise, and is definitely the flavor of the month. The term refers to a connected-ness between the mental and physical processes when engaging in a physical activity. In theory, by engaging in a physical activity one can find a higher level of consciousness. By seeking a higher level of consciousness, in terms of the way we approach our physical activity, we can then achieve a higher level of performance. More often than not, proponents of the mind/body connection tend to refer to the mind and the body as two separate entities. I tend to think of this concept in a more holistic or all-encompassing manner. I personally believe that the mind and the body cannot be separated, as they are parts of a whole. By enabling these two disparate parts of our persona to cooperate towards achieving a common goal, we are capable of exceeding our limitations. When the mind and the body are working in harmony to support and inspire one another, and are actively involved in achieving a shared objective, we are perhaps living our lives at the highest possible level. Living at this heightened level is really the point of this book.

In the context of Hot Point Fitness, there are a number of techniques that you can utilize to heighten communication between the mind and the body. Much like transforming our physical appearance, improving our mental performance must be seen as a journey. It is not something that will happen overnight, but it is something that can be developed rapidly. This chapter will outline five strategies to help you on this journey. The five steps are: to set reasonable goals, to commit yourself to the journey, to dedicate a prescribed amount of time to get to that destination, to give 100% of your effort, and to focus your mind completely on the task at hand.

Set Your Goals

You deserve the greatest opportunity to realize your dreams. Setting goals is the greatest tool you can have to become successful. There are many ways to set your goals, and many aids that may be used along the journey to keep yourself motivated and moving forward. When creating a goal, you must, above all else, be reasonable. As you begin, you may want to set goals that can reasonably be achieved. In achieving those goals, you can feel triumphant. You can gain esteem, you can feel that you are ready for the challenge, you can be catapulted towards the next conquest. If, however, you set your goals too high, you may defeated; you may feel like a failure. In setting goals, you are attempting to reinforce the positive, to promote self-love. Set yourself up to excel. Set yourself up to succeed. The idea is to create an aura of achievement around this one activity in your life, and to enable that achievement to have profound ramifications in every aspect of your life.

The first and most important thing to focus on is a long-term goal. What motivated you to buy this book, and what is it, exactly, that you would like to see change? This is a huge question, and there may be some emotional baggage that comes with this answer. I have had many people come to me with the hope that I could help them to lose a substantial amount of fat. Although many of my clients have come for this reason, one person, in particular, stands out as an example of the issues that I want to touch upon.

Donna was not always heavy, but after the tragic death of her husband and child, she began to gain weight at a rapid pace. The more she gained, the less frequently she left her home. When she came in to see me, it was the first time she had left her house in many months, and she was not able to walk without the aid of canes to support her weight. On some level, I could sense that she was almost giving up on life, and that coming to see me might have been her way to fight against that downward spiral. Although she told me that all she wanted was to lose some weight, what was really happening was that she was desperately trying to say "yes" to life again. Although this is an extreme example, we all have underlying issues and motivations. Be mindful to pinpoint yours.

When you are able to pinpoint what it is you want to change about your body, stop to consider what may have caused the condition in the first place. I would also like you to spend some time pondering what that change would mean for you—what it would look like, how it would feel, and how it would change your life. The woman that I mentioned earlier did, in fact, lose a substantial amount of weight. As a point of reference, she lost over 135 pounds of *fat*. Not only is she able to walk without the aid of her canes but she is now training for a marathon. People who have known her for years do not recognize her on the street. To her, this transformation has not only meant that she is leaner and healthier but that she is comfortable leaving her home, she is enjoying social activities, has enough energy to do things for others, and that she is feeling passionate about living again. Through her process of transformation, she was able to bring closure to the losses in her life. By doing that, she was able to go on living, and living passionately. I am not saying that I had much, if anything, to do with that process. I am only saying that setting up an avenue for those changes to occur helped her reach an emotional destination that was far more profound than weight loss. I would like you to visualize what the changes you desire may bring to you in terms of added benefits. Really spend the time visualizing these changes in your mind's eye. Would you have a better relationship with your spouse or loved one? Would people feel that you are more open to them? Would people find you more attractive? Would you recapture some lost vitality? Would you feel more alive? This is not a lesson in daydreaming. It is an exercise in visualization. It is an exercise for your will. It is the process of informing your body—by way of the mind—what you really want.

When the mind and the body are working in unison and harmony, it is possible to achieve the unimaginable. At one time or another, we have all felt like we wanted to change the world. In transforming your body, you are beginning with yourself first. You will soon understand how this transformation will impact the world around you. To transform your physical body, you will place certain expectations upon yourself. These expectations will emphasize qualities that plant the seeds for success and can only be seen as positive. In reading this book and following the program set forth within these covers, you are committing yourself to becoming the best that you can be, and, on some level, to passionately live up to your potential.

I have asked you to spend some time visualizing what this destination would look and feel like for you. We have defined this as your ultimate long-term goal, your destination. While merely visualizing this change will not get you to your destination, I have several suggestions to bridge the gap from where you are right now to that place you want to get to. What I am suggesting is that you create a series of landmarks to mark your path along your journey. While you were reading the first chapter, you made a promise to yourself that you will spend at least one hour of your day, three times a week, achieving excellence. That promise is the first of these landmarks. This first landmark is a commitment to begin the journey of transformation. As you recall, I asked only that you try this for two weeks. Having made that commitment, you made a short-term goal. You may have to make several of these over the next two weeks. You may make a short-term goal to even show up for your commitment. Once you meet that goal, you may make a promise to yourself that you will finish your entire time allotment for your aerobic exercise—another short-term goal. You may be asked out for dinner, and you will look yourself in the mirror and promise yourself that you will stick to your nutrition program for that meal—yet another short-term goal. You may decide that your short-term goal is to reach Phase Three of the Hot Point Program . . . you may create a short-term goal of just doing one repetition of one exercise to perfection. It does not matter how small your goals are, it only matters that you set them and then meet them. If we try to live in the past, we will fail by reliving all of our mistakes. If we try to live in the future, we will never get there, because we will be living a dream. You can only reach your dream by living in the present and working towards that dream, that final destination . . . your ultimate goal. Each and every day that you spend working with Hot Point Fitness, you will have created and met literally hundreds of goals during your workout. You will see that this creates momentum, a force of positive achievement, and the self-satisfaction of a job well done.

Commit to the Journey

Realize your transformation will require your commitment to persevere. Your commitment will be tested often, and there are a number of ways to prevent giving in to them. Perseverance means to not let anything, and I mean anything, prevent you from realizing your goal. And there will be many things that get in your way. External things like weather, car trouble, cold and flu season, feeling tired, or feeling sad . . . Believe me, you will come up with thousands of excuses. Overcome those reasons not to be what you are dreaming to be. You have seen, in your mind's eye, what it would be like to realize your goal. So I ask you, how bad do you want it? The greater your desire, the greater your ability to overcome the obstacle that could get in your way. Want it! Get yourself to your workout. Drag yourself there kicking and screaming if you have to, but get yourself to at least show up.

There are many games we play to get ourselves to do something we may not want to do. Simple things like saying, "I should." Many people reward themselves for doing the things they do not really want to do. Some people guilt themselves into doing it . . . "If I don't do it, then I'll feel horrible." Personally, I stand by commitments when it costs me something. If there are consequences if I fail to honor my commitments, then I usually stand by them. If I actually pay for something, I want to get my money's worth. If you really want to transform your body, plunk down some hard-earned money and join a gym. Aside from having a place to go with all the equipment you need and want, you will be placing yourself in an environment with many people who share similar goals. Joining a gym also eliminates a whole host of excuses and distractions.

Set Aside Time

You will not have achieved your ultimate goal after your first workout. Your transformation will take time. You must carve out a predetermined amount of time during your day, and be consistent in this time commitment. You must commit yourself to the journey, and once committed you will begin seeing profound results, and find yourself becoming even more dedicated to achieving your ultimate goal. Think of this time, the time you have set aside for your transformation, as your sanctuary or a safe haven. Look upon this time as if it were a part of your day that provides a vacation from the rest of your life. This time is to be spent building yourself up physically, mentally, and emotionally. You can regain lost property and lost money, but it is never possible to regain time. This is the one commodity that is most valuable in our lives. You are investing this prescribed amount of time to reap the profits associated with the investment.

100% Effort & Focus

As you are investing the most important commodity you possess, time, it is essential that you maximize your effort during that precious time. Whether you are just beginning this process or you have lifted weights and exercised for years, it is essential that you learn and relearn the concepts and basics to both do the Hot Point exercises properly and achieve the maximum result for your effort. To perform the Hot Point exercises properly requires you to execute them with perfect or nearly perfect technique. To execute perfection demands focus. This acute focus is almost like tunnel vision. The room around you will virtually disappear, and the more you can focus on the precision of the movement, the greater the depth of your experience. The greater this focus becomes, the closer you come to giving this workout, this time, this goal, 100% of your effort.

Many who routinely exercise come into the gym and are fairly unconscious about what they are doing. They go in for an hour or longer, they do their aerobic exercise, they lift their weights, and they are frustrated that they are not getting the results they want. The problem is not that exercise isn't working, the problem is that they are not doing the exercises in a manner that maximizes the effort, and they are not engaging their mind in the process.

The journey is both external and internal. Although others may not notice this internal change, your resolve has already changed you from within. As you reach your goals, you will be motivated to attain greater achievements, and those will give rise to even greater ones. You will see positive changes in your personal and professional relationships, in your job performance, and in the way you are maximizing your time. You will find you are capable of doing more, of having more, of enjoying more. You will have far less stress, your health will be vastly improved, you will feel infinitely better about yourself, and you will have the energy to live your life joyously and passionately. As you become the master of your own body, you are giving yourself the tools needed to become master of your destiny.

The Mental Game

If you have ever watched televised sports, you are not unfamiliar with terms like "mental toughness," or hearing the announcer refer to a superstar athlete as "the most intelligent player to play the game," or an athlete having a "mental lapse." If you play a sport, you know firsthand that the physical aspect of the game is only half of the picture. Skilled players can become excellent players merely by making a mental adjustment, and excellent players can become superstars by improving their mental game. With Hot Point Fitness, you will be attempting to take your workout to a higher level, and this requires that you improve your mental game. Whether you have been in training for years or working out is a new concept to you, mental preparation, mental clarity, and mental focus are essential to derive the maximum benefit from this work.

Mental conditioning is perhaps the most fundamental factor of this program. It is how well you use your brain that will determine if you succeed or fail both on this program and in your life. For our purposes, this mental conditioning will take two forms: using our heads to keep our bodies challenged, and using our imaginative skills to help us achieve real and tangible goals.

There are people who have trained for years without the results that are commensurate with their effort. This phenomenon is referred to as a training plateau. If you go to the gym often, you may see the same person on the treadmill next to you each morning. They may have been next to you every morning for years, and yet they do not look any different than the first time you saw them. They are stuck at a certain training level and cannot get out of the rut no matter how many times a week they go to the gym. Whether you are new to exercise or have been exercising for years, it is essential to employ the mind to avoid this syndrome.

The body is a resilient, efficient, and highly intelligent entity. When people reach a training plateau, or observe that the results they are working so hard to achieve begin to slow or even stop, it means that our innate ability to adapt to stress and physical demands has been activated and has allowed the body to shift into something like "cruise control." In fact, there are "granola" or esoteric principles such as muscular memory at work, meaning that your body knows exactly what will be asked of it and will expend only the minimal amount of energy to complete the task. To achieve the results you desire will necessitate that you out-think your body, shock it, surprise it, and keep it guessing.

The reason why people can exercise for years without significant results is because they are locked into a routine. Each time they go to the gym, they are doing exactly the same thing, in the same order. The body knows what is coming and can just tune out and go through the motions. This is mindless exercise; exercise becomes a regimen that you *do not* want to adhere to. The object of *this* exercise is to be creative . . . to never do the same workout twice. Look at the average man or woman who runs a marathon. Do they look like they are extremely fit? Are they a little flabby? Is their musculature well defined? Do they look especially healthy? The answer is most probably, "No." These men and women train continuously, and their bodies have become quite used to the demands. Because the body is a resilient and self-sustaining entity, even while these athletes are expending terrific amounts of energy, their bodies insist on conserving as much as they possibly can. As a consequence, these athletes are not highly developed physically. Think about how many miles a week these athletes run. If you expended that amount of energy, how would you like to look? The creativity you bring to your workout makes all the difference. For instance, if you are training with weights, and working on three individual muscle groups that day, there are several exercises for each muscle group. If you do these exercises in a particular order, and never stray from the routine, you will consequently never achieve the results you desire. If, however, you change the order of exercises for each muscle group, and/or change the order of muscle groups you are working on so that you do not replicate two consecutive workouts, the body will not know what is coming next and will develop at a more accelerated rate. Much of your success is predicated on this element of surprise. By using your creativity to outthink the body, you can maximize your effort tremendously. Utilizing your creativity in this way will also ensure that you never become bored and will continually be challenged both mentally and physically.

Mental Preparation

Mental preparation is a significant factor in maximizing your effort. I have watched players take the field long before the rest of the team begins warming up. They visualize their every move and "see" the game before it even starts. One of my most physically successful clients spends fifteen minutes alone in the locker room visualizing the workout he is about to undertake. He is the most focused person I have ever seen in a gym. He has a purpose. There is nothing that can distract him. There is nothing that will stop him from achieving his goals. After employing this technique in the gym, I really wanted to test this theory.

I am a terrible golfer. I have probably played the game three times in my life. I haven't played for several years, but was invited to play the other day with some clients. Before I began, I visualized the course and visualized myself swinging the club effortlessly and hitting the ball straight, which were, incidentally, things I was not yet able to do anywhere but in my fantasies. The last time I played, it is possible that I was secretly banned from all golf courses in the area and labeled "a hazard to others." However, after visualizing my game and remaining focused throughout the afternoon, I was shocked to look down at my scorecard to discover I had broken 80. The moral of the story is that exercising should not be mindless. When you can set your mind to the work, you can increase your results dramatically. Yes, there are limits to your physical capability, but employing your mind may indeed enable you to surpass those limitations.

You must train yourself to visualize the goal before you can actually attain it. If I have a client attempting to lift a particularly heavy weight, I will ask them to close their eyes and visualize themselves doing the entire set. Once they have completed that visualization, they will open their eyes, I will count to three, and they will complete the set. They are able to achieve something they may not have thought attainable because they have "seen" themselves accomplish the task. If you were working as a secretary, and really wanted to be the CEO of the company, you would first have to imagine yourself attaining that post before you could even contemplate climbing your way up the corporate ladder. The image of yourself in that position could indeed motivate and propel you to higher and higher levels. The same is true of physical transformation. Harnessing and using your creativity to visualize your goals and to meditate upon them regularly will accelerate the process of attaining those goals and pave the road to success.

As you progress, you will be increasing the number of days you exercise, or the time you spend doing aerobic exercise, reducing the amount of calories you take in, or the amount of weight you are lifting. All of these variables are adjusted incrementally and will require mental adjustments to meet the challenge each presents to you. We are talking about small changes, but these small changes are often the difference between victory and defeat. I recently read a study polling real estate agents who were once making $80,000 and are now making in excess of

$1,000,000. When asked what it was they were doing differently, they all had an almost identical reply. Essentially they all were doing just about the same thing as before. They just increased their effort about 10% across the board. They increased their productivity in many different areas by only a small amount, and yet their bottom-line return was astounding. The same principle will be applicable to you and this workout. It is the difference between quitting your aerobics early and staying on the treadmill an extra five minutes. It is the difference of doing those last three reps when you are really tired. It is the difference between having French fries or a salad. It is just that final push, that last little bit of effort, that builds your confidence level, your self-esteem, and makes you know that you have achieved excellence. Giving it your best, your all, is the feeling that stokes the fire of desire. Feeling that you went all out in the effort is what makes you know you can live your dream. Giving your all is what makes the victory taste so sweet. The difference between 90% of your effort and 100% of your effort will mean having your dream within your grasp or living the joy of your dream. It is giving an additional 10% across the board, and doing it consistently, that will bring you closer and closer to your ultimate goal. While you will be practicing "giving it your all" in the gym at least three days a week, you will soon realize that this concept can be taken out of the gym and applied to your everyday life with profound, life-changing results.

3

The Hot Point Pyramid
of Understanding

Aerobics, Weight Training and Eating to Win

By now it should be clear that you will derive a wealth of benefits from regular exercise, and I can't emphasize enough the importance of your desire, your will, your commitment, and how your mental preparation will ultimately help you to realize your transformation. It is now time to put that information into the context of this transformational work. Hot Point Fitness is a process to dramatically transform your body. Not only is Hot Point Fitness a method to completely redesign the way your body looks, but it is also an avenue to transform the way you feel and also the way you feel about yourself.

Hot Point Fitness is built on the premise of three basic principles. If you want to get leaner and become fit, there are only three things that you can do, and three things only. I call these three principles the pyramid of understanding. On this program, you will be utilizing weight training, nutrition, and aerobic training as a three-pronged attack to reach your ultimate goal. Think of weight training, nutrition, and aerobic training as the three sides of the pyramid. If the foundation were not in place, there would be nothing to support the walls. If one of the two walls were not in place, the pyramid would collapse in on itself. The same is true of your transformation. Weight training, nutrition, and aerobics must be in place for the transformation to occur. Once the transformation occurs, these three elements have to remain in place, or your pyramid may eventually crumble under the sands of time.

It is the manner in which you build these three sides of the pyramid that will ultimately determine the strength of the entire structure. If you do indeed want to transform your body, it is imperative that you incorporate aerobic exercise, weight training, and nutrition into a comprehensive program. To define and create tone throughout the musculature of your body, you will be implementing the most revolutionary and scientifically based resistance training program ever devised. This effort is supported by what goes into your body (your diet), and also by the additional activity you will perform to burn off the food that you eat (aerobic activity). It is the strength of your aerobic regimen, the efficiency of your weight training routine, and the effectiveness of your diet that determine your results.

If you do any one of the three, you will enjoy modest health benefits and may improve your level of fitness or reduce the fat on your body by a small percentage. If you were to do two of the three, you would see only moderate improvement in these areas. If, however, you were to incorporate all three strategies, you could have tremendous success. If you did not use all three, it could take a very long time to realize these changes. There may be extended periods of time when your results would plateau, and you could be stuck in a rut indefinitely. It is the manner in which you perform your aerobic and weight training exercises, and how effective your nutrition program is, that spell success or failure. If you could incorporate all three strategies (aerobics, weight training, and nutrition) into a comprehensive program that is designed to maximize each activity, you will not only possess a recipe for success, but you will be able to reach your goals in a very time-efficient manner. The combining of these three vital ingredients is the premise of Hot Point Fitness.

There have been many books devoted to the three sides of your pyramid. There is enough information available on weight training, aerobic training and cardiovascular work, and diet to fill entire libraries. In this wealth of available information, there are many viewpoints and often there are conflicting opinions as to what the most effective strategy actually is. The problem with much of this information is that it has not been proved to be effective. In fact, much of the information available on these subjects will often be counterproductive for you. Since the

1970s, the worlds of physical fitness and nutrition have gone through an evolutionary process. And little by little, information surfaces that turns previously held convictions upside down. I personally believe that the fields of fitness and nutrition are presently in need of some breakthrough information that will cause revolutionary changes. In providing you with what I have found to be the most effective strategies for weight training, aerobic training, and nutrition, it is my hope that you will be armed with precisely that kind of revolutionary information.

The premise of Hot Point is to create a new paradigm for fitness. The word paradigm, or paradigm shift, is often associated with technological advances, such as the Internet or "new economy" stocks. Something new comes along, something that people were not expecting, and we can never turn back to the way things were before. In essence, that new thing changes every notion or thought we have had on any particular subject. Hot Point Fitness creates the most scientifically sound principles for weight training and combines these principles with effective strategies for nutrition and aerobic training. It then combines these three winning strategies into a comprehensive program to get the greatest results for your effort, to achieve your goals quickly, and do so in a time-efficient manner.

The objective is to have the old you melt into the new you that you are working so diligently to create. The point of Hot Point Weight Training is to work each muscle to 100% of its capacity, and consequently completely transform the way the muscles in your body look. The point of Hot Point Nutrition is to speed the metabolism and make it burn calories at a white-hot pace. Hot Point Aerobics will superheat your muscles and burn fat from your body quickly, safely, and forever. When all three strategies are combined to fulfill a personal goal, there is no obstacle that cannot be overcome, and no goal that is out of reach. What are your goals, and how dramatic is the transformation you are seeking? No matter where you are right at this moment, no matter where you would like to get, no matter how old you are, no matter when you last exercised regularly, Hot Point Fitness will be the road map to your destination.

When I first meet with a client, often times they do not express a clear goal, but simply say, "I just want to look better." After working together for a short period of time, "looking better" becomes more defined. A winning strategy for resistance training sets in motion a series of positive events, and obstacles are overcome like falling dominoes. The strategy for nutrition and the consistency of aerobic training program dictate how quickly results are achieved. To deepen your understanding of the pyramid, you need to understand how a program that utilizes weight training, nutrition, and aerobic exercise is the fastest and safest way to achieve your goals.

Weight training is *the* vital ingredient in your transformation. Weight training has the greatest ability to transform your appearance, to shape and define the muscles in your body, to create a balanced appearance, and also to positively alter your metabolism. Most people, especially women, shy away from weight training. Have no fear. If done correctly, weight training will not make you muscle-bound, restrict your motion, or eventually turn to fat. These are all misconceptions. Weight training will create definition in the muscle, lead to more muscle density, help your body eliminate fat, and will ultimately help you to look the way you really want to look.

As most people are not working out to compete in bodybuilding contests, nor do they have any desire to look like a bodybuilder, the goal of weight training is not to simply build muscular bulk but to create beautiful elongated musculature throughout your body. In essence the goal is to create *density* in the musculature, not mass. There is a great difference between density and mass. Mass is simply the size or how big any particular muscle is, whereas muscle density refers to the amount and number of fibers within the muscle. I am not particularly large. When I am wearing street clothes, you wouldn't be able to tell that I am able to lift greater weights than most of the bodybuilders at the gym. The secret of strength is in the density, not the size of the muscle. To further promote the creation of muscle density in each muscle group that you work, there is a corresponding stretch for those muscles. This not only increases flexibility but also allows the muscle to heal more quickly, thereby creating muscle density and promoting the development of elongated musculature. To achieve the greatest results in the shortest amount of time requires a support system for your weight training. While it is scientifically proven that increasing muscle density speeds the metabolism, your transformation is only possible with the help of diet and aerobic activity.

Next to resistance training, the most important facet of the program is creating a nutritional program that works for you. Diet could be considered the foundation of the pyramid, a constant upon which your transformation rests. When people say, "I want to look better," they are most often talking about losing some weight. Let's first dismiss some notions about weight loss. On this program you will be burning off *fat*. Weight is irrelevant. Fat is what should be counted. On this program it is essential that you know precisely how much fat you have. To create the proper formula to reach your goals and also to gauge your progress, you must have your

HOT POINT FITNESS

body-fat percentage measured. When you have this measurement taken, you will discover two very valuable pieces of information. The first and most valuable piece of information will be how much lean muscle mass you have. This amount of lean muscle mass is exactly what you are striving to have more of. Based upon the amount of lean muscle mass, you can determine how much you need to eat. It is precisely this lean muscle mass that you want to feed. The second piece of information is how much fat you are carrying around with you. This is the stuff you want to lose. If you want to have a washboard stomach, I can promise you that you already have it, but the problem is that there is fat covering up the muscle and you can't see it. Since we want to lose this fat, and we do not want more of it, we must not provide the fat with food.

As an example, let's look at two identical female twins. They are identical in every way. They weigh exactly the same; they have exactly the same goals. Twin #1 goes on a restrictive diet. Twin #2 buys this book and utilizes aerobics, resistance training, and proper nutrition to transform her physical appearance. She has her body-fat percentage taken before she begins and takes measurements so that she knows which limbs are larger than others. She can then determine where she wants to lose and gain inches. Twin #1 "just wants to lose some weight." After two weeks on her restrictive diet, she weighs herself on the scale and discovers she has lost five pounds. By depriving herself, Twin #1 did drop 5 pounds, but lost those pounds in water weight, muscle, and bone density. Because she has lost muscle and bone density, she now actually has a greater percentage of fat than when she started. Conversely, after the same two weeks, Twin #2 weighs herself and finds she has lost 3 pounds. She has her body-fat percentage measured and is told that she has lost five pounds of fat and gained two pounds of muscle and bone density. Twin #2 added lean muscle mass, and that is exactly what fuels the body to burn fat. She has set herself up to burn off even more fat in her next two weeks on the program, and people are already noticing the physical changes in her appearance. The bottom line is that Twin #1 looks pretty much the same, but Twin #2 has dropped a dress size.

Aerobic exercise is also very important. It not only is beneficial for your heart, circulation, and overall health but it is the key ingredient to burning off excess calories and then eventually burning off fat. If you already go to the gym, you may have seen others really struggling with aerobic exercise. They may really push themselves and see no results. The truth of the matter is that you really only need to perform aerobic exercise for a relatively small amount of time to achieve the maximum result. There is a performance window that you will formulate that insures that you are getting the most return for your investment of time. After just a few weeks, this form of exercise will not exhaust you but, conversely, will get all of the endomorphs flowing and actually boost your energy level. There are many exercises you can perform to get an aerobic workout. It will take some experimentation to determine what suits you best, but this form of exercise will ultimately be the most rewarding and addictive activity for you.

When these three elements, aerobic activity, weight training, and nutrition, are put together into a comprehensive program, your results are guaranteed. Through weight training, you will be developing and defining the musculature—adding lean muscle mass and decreasing your body-fat percentage. By implementing a sound nutritional program, you will be feeding only that lean muscle and burning off fat. By engaging in aerobic exercise, you will improve your circulation, strengthen your heart, increase your endurance, become more physically fit, and most importantly, you will be using stored fat to fuel your activity. When all three of these elements are in place, there is nothing—***absolutely nothing***—that can prevent you from attaining your ultimate goal.

By bringing all three elements of the pyramid together, you create a certain momentum. Your nutritional program supports your aerobic training efforts. Your weight training will support your aerobic activity. Your weight training affects your diet. It is like *The Little Engine That Could*. You chug, chug, chug up the hill saying, "I think I can, I think I can." And with each turn of the wheel, the three elements of your transformation take hold. You begin feeling the changes . . . seeing the changes when you look in the mirror. Suddenly, there is momentum. And your aerobic training, weight training, and diet are all working to complement each other. You see the top of the hill. You begin chanting, "I know I can, I know I can," as you reach the top. Then something magical happens. You begin coasting downhill. You do not have to work as hard, but your transformation unfolds at rapid pace. Faster and faster changes are occurring, dramatically affecting the way you look and feel. You then just have to keep the train on the tracks.

There are three levels in Hot Point Fitness, and they represent landmarks that act as a gateway to a new level of fitness and commitment. These three landmarks are called Phase One, Phase Two, and Phase Three. In Phase One you will be spending one hour at the gym, three days per week. Phase One is designed simply to incorporate exercise and proper nutrition into your life. This stage will increase in difficulty as your hunger for challenge increases. The point of Phase One is for you to make exercise a habit, to learn to depend on exercise to relieve stress, to be something that you look forward to doing, to increase your activity level, and to get you nearer to your goals. I have many clients who exercise at this level and are very comfortable. This level is recommended for those that have hectic work schedules, for those who want a moderate level of fitness, or for those who are beginning this journey.

In Phase Two you will be spending 90 minutes at the gym four days per week. In Phase Two the habit that you've formed turns into an addiction. You form a dependency on exercise to keep your spirits lifted, and if you miss one of your sessions, you will actually feel sluggish and lethargic. You will also accelerate the pace of your results and find yourself coming closer and closer to achieving your ultimate goal. This phase is ideal for those who are fairly active and are looking for substantial change. After just a short time, you will feel your body changing gears and shifting into overdrive.

In Phase Three you can spend up to two hours a day at the gym, five days per week. Phase Three is the level that I train my clients who are professional athletes. I will take you through the exact workout that they do. Although this level of fitness is not the exclusive domain of professional athletes, it is extremely rigorous. And if you can get yourself into this phase, you will certainly be more fit that 95% of the general public. When you achieve this level of fitness, you can call yourself a Hot Point Junkie, as there is no higher level to this addiction. You will need it. You will crave it. You will do everything you can to maintain your addiction and all the amazing benefits that this addiction gives to you. Of course, you can stay within any of these three phases for as long as you like. Conceivably, you could stay in any one of the three phases for the rest of your life. It all depends on how much time you want to devote to your transformation, and what your ultimate goal is. Hot Point Training is the road map to take you to your destination.

It is absolutely essential that the three sides of your pyramid be sound. You are building a structure for the ages. You are building a structure that must hold up against the sands of time. You are building a temple. So important are these three principles that I would like to discuss them in great detail over the next three chapters. No matter what level of exercise you currently enjoy, whether you are just beginning or have practiced these three disciplines all your life, it is essential that you read the next three chapters. If you are just beginning, use the next three chapters as if they were a one-on-one session with your personal trainer. Over the next three chapters, you will learn the philosophy and the scientific principles that are the basis for your transformation. If you have been exercising for years, the next three chapters will be equally valuable, perhaps even more so. No matter how much you think you might know about the subject, attempt to rethink your currently held convictions on these subjects and completely alter what you are currently practicing. Over the next three chapters, you will pick up a few precious gems that will take your level of fitness to heights previously unknown to you. These chapters on aerobics, weight training, and nutrition are the three sides of the pyramid, the strongest and most wondrous structure that man has ever known. It is time to learn the real secrets of pyramid power.

4

Create Muscle Strength at a Deeper Level . . . Quickly

Hot Point Momentum-less Resistance Training

Resistance training, commonly known as weight training, is one of the most misunderstood and maligned forms of exercise. Given the many misconceptions surrounding weight training, fear often replaces reason for would-be enthusiasts. Many people look at weight training with skepticism, fear, or disdain. Many women are hesitant to exercise with weights for fear that they will get muscle-bound, or look manly as a result of the process. The elderly sometimes fear that weight training will somehow injure them. Many people who are overweight fear that weight training will only make them bigger. Nothing could be further from the truth. Proper weight training will increase the density of your muscle, increasing the amount of lean muscle mass. Weight training is the most effective means to create lean muscle mass and change our appearance. Lean muscle mass is the greatest asset we can have. By increasing our lean muscle mass, we automatically reduce the percentage of fat we are carrying around with us. Lean muscle mass burns more calories than fat, and helps our body process the food that we eat more efficiently. When our bodies are working more efficiently, we experience higher levels of energy throughout the day. We accelerate our metabolism and boost our immune systems. Weight training also builds, tones, or firms up muscle. Rather than making you look "manly," weight training can make women look even more feminine, by creating muscular definition in just the right places, and accentuating the natural curves of your body. As we age, we naturally lose lean muscle mass. If you are elderly, you do not have to lift a great amount of weight to derive all the benefits . . . you can use small amounts of weight to build your muscles back up to where they used to be when you were younger. Many clients I have trained are retirement age and older. They have told me repeatedly that weight training has actually offset the aging process. They feel confident in their movement, they have regained a sense of strength, flexibility, and balance that they thought was gone forever. And, I have seen literally hundreds of people who were extremely overweight have unbelievable success with weight training.

They say that beauty is only skin deep. I tend to disagree. It is precisely what is going on underneath the skin that can be so beautiful. Very few people exercise to get healthier. Most of us exercise to look fantastic. So let's not try to fool each other. What you are striving to accomplish is a complete physical transformation. By even attempting to embark on this journey, overwhelming changes will begin to take hold. You will bolster your confidence, raise your energy level, elevate your self-esteem, heighten your sense of accomplishment, and alter forever the manner in which you approach your life and the people you encounter. In the process of transformation, you will find no greater ally than the Hot Point Weight Training System.

I began perfecting the Hot Point Weight Training System over fifteen years ago, while I was still in college. As part of my education, I wanted to scientifically determine if weight training was truly a viable form of exercise to get in top physical condition. If it was, I also wanted to find out why some people trained for many years without significant results. I began by studying the exercises that were practiced by athletes and bodybuilders adhering to a strict weight-training regimen. I became more and more puzzled. The exercises seemed to be targeting all the necessary muscle groups, but an extremely large percentage of people failed to see changes. These people were putting in a great deal of time and effort, but not getting the results.

As part of my research, I studied the body using the most experimental and technologically advanced magnetic resonance imaging available. With this advanced MRI technology, one can see exactly which muscles are at work during exercise. I also used an infrared image, where the heat given off by the body is seen in terms of color. For each several degrees in temperature, the infrared shows a different color. From black to white, with a spectrum of color in between, one can clearly see which portion of each muscle is working the hardest. It was apparent where the muscle was being optimized, as it appeared to become "*hot*" on the image. I began to focus on this "hot" area of the muscle, both as a beacon of hope that total transformation was possible, and also as a foundation of information to build from.

After studying these images, I was astounded to discover that what you may know as traditional weight-training exercises largely failed to successfully isolate a particular muscle group and work it to its full potential. Instead, traditional weight-training exercises only work 20% to 30% of the targeted muscles. No wonder these athletes were not experiencing more dramatic results! Even if they had worked five times harder, or did the impossible by lifting five times more per week, they could not have achieved significant results. The MRI images proved to me that their traditional weight training was affecting only 30% of the muscle. In other words, the exercises that most people were performing were only affecting the top third of the muscle nearest the skin. The challenge was to reach the 70% of the muscle that was not affected. Through this study, I became quite certain that weight training was still a very viable means to develop musculature, but there were inherent problems with the manner in which people were going about it. I came to the conclusion that there had to be a better way to train the body.

I began to look at the muscular structure for possible answers. I soon learned that our muscle tissue is an ever-changing entity. Seen in the light of physical transformation, muscle tissue, or lean muscle mass, is a most beneficial asset. Lean muscle mass offsets the amount of fat we have on our bodies, boosts our metabolism, and even at rest will burn calories at a high rate. This muscle tissue is also capable of almost infinite growth. Muscle tissue is made up of myriad fibers. When you work a muscle, the fibers that make up the muscle will tear on a microscopic level. If you have ever performed a series of exercises you were not used to, it is precisely this tearing (coupled with lactic acid) that makes you feel sore the next day. This microscopic tearing then heals, creating muscle fibers that are denser than before. This density does not necessarily mean that the muscle gets larger. When you create muscular density, it only means that more fibers exist within the same space. This muscular density occurs exponentially for a very long time before the size of the muscle actually increases. Knowing this, I felt that if I could develop a system to work the muscle from its deepest point all the way to the surface, the results would be astounding.

Using all the anatomical information available to me, I focused on the way in which the muscle was attached to the body, and how the muscle helps, allows, and enables us to move. I compared these observations to our popular notions of exercise. After determining that traditional exercises were clearly invented to work particular parts of the body, I began to test their effectiveness. I quickly came to the conclusion that exercises which relied on resistance or depended on moving weight had the greatest potential to tap into the 70% of our physical potential that was not being used. I found that by altering existing exercises or creating entirely new exercises, I was able to develop a system that should work the entirety of the muscle. I could feel the difference when I did these exercises, but I wanted to test these theories for their practical application. I began teaching these new excercises to high-end athletes, and all of them enjoyed dramatic and tremendous gains that they did not think was possible.

This was the birth of "Hot Point Fitness." Through this study, I came to believe that weight training is not only a viable means of exercise but possibly the form of exercise which offers us the most valuable tools to aid in a physical transformation. In the fifteen years since I made this discovery, I have honed and perfected the system. Hot Point Weight Training is designed to work 100% of the muscle, breaking the muscle down at its deepest level. When those microscopic tears heal, they are transforming 100% of the muscle from its deepest point to the point nearest the skin. This means that you will have a very time-efficient workout, you will be able to see results more quickly, and you will truly transform your entire physical appearance. As a personal trainer, I have helped thousands of people reach their goals and completely transform the way they look and feel. Again, whether you are elderly or out of shape, whether you have been lifting weights for years, whether male or female, whether you want to tone up or bulk up, Hot Point Weight Training is the primary form of exercise that will help you to achieve your goals.

When discussing the topic of weight training, we should establish some common vocabulary. In the pages to follow you may hear one or two words you are not familiar with. In the exercises outlined, a specific number of repetitions and a specific number of sets are prescribed. A repetition is the completion of pushing or moving the weight from point A to point B. You will be instructed to perform that particular exercise for a specific number of repetitions. When you have done this, you will have completed a set.

To maximize your effort, and to truly work 100% of the muscle's capability, you'll need to be diligent and you'll need to concentrate. Each exercise in the Hot Point System is designed to isolate a particular and specific muscle or muscle group. Technically, the muscle that you are targeting is called the primary muscle. Sometimes another muscle aids the primary muscle in a movement. This helper is called a secondary muscle. As you'd expect, the secondary muscle will not be working at 100% of its capability for this particular exercise, even though it is in use. Some parts of the body are not autonomous and moving them means that several muscles or even muscle groups are involved in the motion. For example, when you throw a ball, more than just your shoulder is involved in the process. You are also using your legs, the muscles in your back, your chest, your abdominal muscles, etc. These are called tertiary (meaning third) muscles. These muscles are working at an even smaller percentage of their potential than the secondary muscles.

Because it is our goal to isolate the targeted muscle as much as possible, it is essential that you eliminate any extraneous movement. I call this *momentum-less training*.

Momentum-less training means limiting the movement to fully isolate the target muscle. By eliminating any swinging, throwing, or jerking movements while exercising with weights, you insure that the primary muscle is the sole focus of your work. When you swing, throw, or jerk the weight, many other muscles are helping you to perform the exercise. In a sense, you are cheating because you are calling upon the strength of these other muscles. In fact, you are cheating yourself because you will not be maximizing the muscle of focus. Also, you may be cheating yourself out of the next few weeks of progress, as 90% of injuries occur when you swing or jerk the weights. As a trainer, one of my favorite sayings is, "Bring it, don't swing it." In other words, use the targeted muscle or muscles to move the weight. But this is still only half of the exercise.

When most people work out with weights, they only concern themselves with moving the weight from a starting point to the top of that motion, or from point A to point B. It is the manner in which you release this weight back to point A that is the other half of your exercise that needs to be exploited to maximize 100% of the muscle's capability. When you reach point B, you will control the descent of the weight, rather than letting the weight use its momentum to fall back to its original point of origin. This is called the "negative." This negative gravitational force works the muscle in the exact opposite direction. By consciously eliminating unnecessary secondary and tertiary muscle involvement and using the negative portion of the exercise, you will help yourself a great deal in maximizing 100% of your potential.

It is impossible for a muscle to perform at 100% on the first repetition. For the first several repetitions of an exercise, you will not, nor would you want to, work the muscle to 100% of its capability. Instead you will be working your way to a muscular crescendo, a climax of performance, which happens during the last three or four repetitions of the set. These last few repetitions will and should be difficult. You should have a burning sensation, feel as if your muscles do not have enough blood, and it should be taxing to complete them. This is true especially of your last set in a series of exercises working any particular muscle group. When you are performing the first two-thirds of a set of weight-training exercises, you are exercising at an aerobic level. When you enter into and complete the last third of the set, you should be reaching for and attaining an anaerobic level of exercise. You can only sustain performance at an anaerobic level for a very brief period, and then you have to slow down or stop. In the final repetitions of your set, you must strive to hit the anaerobic level. When you do, you will experience a shaking sensation in the muscles being worked, and you will barely be able to complete the set. The shaking of limbs, the burning sensation, the feeling like you will not be able to complete the set is really the point of the exercise. When you reach this anaerobic stage and could see your muscles in an MRI, they would appear to be hot. This hot point is the point at which you are achieving 100% of your muscle's capability. It makes no difference how much weight you are moving. What you are attempting to do is work the muscle into exhaustion, to a point when it is not physically able to do another repetition. In a sense, the first repetitions are a preparation for the last repetitions of the set, and the first two sets a preparation for the last several repetitions of the last set. This is where and when results occur.

REACHING YOUR GOALS

There are a few fundamental principles to achieving your goals, and it is important to understand them before you begin.

Breathing

The most fundamental principle of life is breathing. Breathing is an involuntary reflex, and it is not something most people think about. It is, however, vital in weight training. Breathing is the zen-like aspect of this program. Correct breathing will allow you to pace yourself throughout your workout. Correct breathing is the key to incorporating the mental aspect of this excercise, and is essential to push through those last reps during the last set. To enlist breathing as your ally, exhale as you drive the weight; hold the weight at the top of the movement; and inhale during the negative motion on a count of "one-two-three." Exhale again to move the weight, and perform the exercise in this way for the prescribed number of repetitions. Believe me, breathing in this way will actually help you move the weight. If you were to inhale when you drive the weight, your breath would actually work against you, and you might not be able to do those last repetitions and never get into the Hot Point result zone.

VARY YOUR ROUTINE

Perhaps the greatest mistake you can make, and one almost everyone who exercises makes, is to get into a routine when you exercise. Most people who go to the gym do almost the exact same routine day after day after day. Besides being tremendously boring, it is often the routine itself that is preventing any noticeable progress. The body is well equipped for adversity and even disaster. The body is designed for your survival. It will conserve as much energy as it can whenever it can. When you perform your exercises in the same way every time you work out, the body gets used to that level of exercise and will only expend the minimal amount of energy needed to perform the task.

To avoid hitting a plateau and to get your body to expend the greatest amount of energy possible, it is vital that you vary your workouts. Essentially, you want to outsmart your body. By changing which parts of the body you work on any given day, by changing the amount of weight from set to set, or by changing the order of exercises, you will keep the body in a suprised state. You are constantly surprising it, shocking it, into performing at the highest level possible. By varying your workout routine, you will avoid many of the pitfalls associated with training plateaus and experience the greatest results possible.

Balance

While most of us strive to look better by working out, very few attempt to balance the body. Nature loves nothing more that symmetry, and in nature we find that symmetry is ultimately what makes the natural world so aesthetically beautiful. The same is true of our bodies. We should strive to ensure that the left arm is the same size as the right arm, the left leg the same size as the right leg, the upper half of our body in proportion to the lower half. Most of us have a dominant arm—we are either right-handed or left-handed. This dominant arm does most of our lifting and is used more often. This dominant arm is bigger and stronger than the other arm. When you work your arms and legs, you always want to work to the weaker side. If you can do eight repetitions with the left side, but you can do fifteen with the right side, just do eight with both. Soon the left will be as strong (and also the same size) as the right side, and you will be able to perform fifteen repetitions on each side.

Your upper body should also be in proportion to the lower body. Most men who work out regularly concentrate mostly on their upper bodies. Their primary areas of focus are on the shoulders, chest, and arms. After months or years of the practice, their bodies become disproportionate and resemble the shape of a Y. The next time you are at the gym, look for the guys that are "Brutus" on the top and "Olive Oyl" on the bottom. It can almost be comedic. If they were to pay equal attention to their leg exercises, their bodies would seem like a whole, rather than two separate entities.

STRETCHING

For every action, there is a reaction. When you are training with weights, you are using the exercise to contract a specific muscle or muscle group. After the muscle has performed at such an optimum level, you need to balance the effort by stretching the muscle out. Many people stretch before they warm up their bodies, and often it is this preventative practice that leads to injury. Think of the muscles in your body as if they were taffy. If you stretch taffy when it is cold, it will not move. If the taffy is warm, the taffy can be stretched. Your muscles are very similar. **You should only stretch *after* you have warmed up the muscles**. Because Hot Point Training will superheat your muscles, you have a built-in opportunity to stretch the muscle when it is the most pliable. Some people simply rest between sets when they train with weights, but this isn't beneficial for you. Rather than resting, maximize your time by stretching the muscle you just worked. By stretching the muscle, you will increase the blood flow to the area that just worked so hard, and the stretch becomes a small reward for the muscle. Increased circulation brings needed ingredients such as oxygen, glucose, and other nutrients which nourish the muscle. Stretching the muscle after working it will offset much of the soreness you feel the next day, help to flush lactic acid out of the muscle tissue, prevent injury, and help fully develop the musculature. Aside from rewarding the body, this stretch will also affect your appearance. Stretching helps to create beautiful elongated muscles, rather than small and constricted ones. For each Hot Point exercise, you will also find a corresponding stretch.

Resistance training with active stretching between sets then becomes an aerobic activity. By not resting, the heart rate remains elevated, the metabolic rate continues to accelerate, and your muscles remain active and warm. By utilizing stretching techniques after each set of resistance training, your workout is taken to another level. Most people who lift weights merely rest between sets. This resting allows the heart to slow down and the body to recuperate too much, and after a certain period of time they are able to go back to perform the next set. Aside from wasting your time, this practice of resting does little else. On the other hand, when you are stretching between sets, the body does not slow down significantly, and the muscles continue to work.

WEIGHT TRAINING TIPS

The single most important aspect of weight training is technique. No matter what your goals, you will not be able to attain them without proper and nearly perfect technique. Even if you have trained for a very long time, I remind you that we are talking about a new paradigm for training with weight. The Hot Point goal is to utilize 100% of the muscle's capability, exhaust the muscle or muscle group, stretch it, and then leave it alone—move on to the next until your next session. Achieving this level of performance will require you to follow the directions and photographs here in order to achieve your highest level of performance.

Each individual has different goals, and while it is essential that proper technique be used, these divergent goals boil down to two basic strategies. While some desire to firm up their musculature and create tone and definition, others look forward to adding considerable size to their muscles and creating bulk. You may want a combination of the two. You may want to add size to your legs and merely create some muscle tone in your chest. You may want bigger biceps, to create size in your lateral muscles to accentuate your waist, and to bring definition to your leg muscles. Although the possibilities and combinations are endless, weight training boils down to toning up and bulking up.

The strategies for toning and building bulk are similar. In both instances, you will utilize the techniques discussed in this chapter. There are only three variables—the amount of weight you are moving; the number of repetitions you are moving that weight; and the number of sets for each exercise. The basic strategy for toning muscle is to perform a greater number of repetitions in the set and to work with a light or medium amount of weight. By using a relatively light weight, a greater number of repetitions will be needed to get the burn and exhaust the muscle. You will perform 20 repetitions of the exercise for each set. The strategy for creating a larger muscle is to lift a relatively heavy amount of weight. You should attempt to perform 10–12 repetitions for each set. To develop considerable bulk, the strategy would be to lift an extremely heavy weight 6–8 repititions.

Determining the amount of weight you can or should be moving will take some experimentation. If I were standing by your side as your personal trainer, it would be quite easy for me to gauge what amount of weight you should be working with just by looking at you. Unfortunately, since I cannot be at your side, you will have to determine weight levels on your own. I strongly suggest that you bring this book along with you as your companion when you go to the gym. In the pages that follow, you will see all the exercises that you will encounter while utilizing the Hot Point Program. If I were at your side as your personal trainer, I would demonstrate the proper technique for each exercise before you attempted it. I often demonstrate these exercises for many months, although my clients have performed the exercises numerous times. Even if you have been exercising with weights for years, I strongly recommend that you utilize the directions to improve your technique each time you work out. Simply follow these directions using a weight that you feel comfortable with. Use your everyday life as a guidepost for this experimentation. (If you have picked up a gallon of milk, you know that you can safely lift ten pounds.) Choose the lightest possible weight for the first repetition, just to get the fundamental technique of the exercise. After you are certain of the proper technique, increase the weight incrementally, until you feel like you would be challenged by performing a set of ten repetitions. Perform ten repetitions of each exercise, and make a notation of the weight in the space provided. This will be your starting point. From here, your transformation begins.

HOT POINT RESISTANCE TRAINING

THE EXERCISES

HOT POINT COMMANDMENTS

1. Always read the description of the exercise before your first set.
2. Visualize the exercise before you perform it.
3. Momentum-less training means "Bring it, don't swing it!"
4. Breathe out to move weight. Breathe in on the negative movement of the exercise.
5. Use proper technique from beginning to end.
6. Stretch between every set for at least 30 seconds.
7. DO NOT break between sets and exercises for longer than one minute.
8. Never perform the exact same workout two days in a row.
9. Wait at least 90 minutes after eating before you work out.
10. Avoid distractions. This is your time!

YOUR LEGS

Your legs are made up of many different muscles and muscle groups. So many, in fact, that if I went into an anatomical description of each and every muscle, it would take up the better part of this book. Suffice it to say that the largest muscles in your body are from the waist down. I stress the legs not only because there are so many muscles but because working the legs properly will improve results in every area of your body. There is no known scientific reason for this, nor have I seen a study that delves into this phenomenon. Perhaps it is caused by the sheer mass of the muscles. Perhaps by increasing the density of these muscles, a chain reaction is sparked throughout the body, promoting growth and stimulating the metabolism. There are many hypotheses, but no one knows for certain. I can only tell you that from my own personal experience, and from the experiences of all the people who I have trained, this much is true: **The more time you spend working the muscles in your legs, the greater your overall level of fitness.**

As with any resistance exercise, it is important to measure your limbs to promote balance before you begin the process of regular weight training. You should measure your thighs at the point nearest your crotch on both sides. You should measure the middle of your thighs at the exact same point, and you should also measure your calves. It is quite normal that one leg is wider in one, if not all, of these measurement spots. In other words, most people have a dominant leg. But to promote balance, and to create the most beautiful aesthetic look, it is essential that both legs be the same size. So if yours aren't, I recommend that you do the following exercises one leg at a time. Each leg should be worked using the same amount of weight and the same number of repetitions. In this way, you will be working to the weaker side. Soon both legs will not only be capable of the exact same demands, but soon they will also be the same size. Remember, the point of all this is to promote balance.

Leg exercises can sometimes be tricky, and if performed incorrectly can cause injury. The joints of your legs will be performing weight-bearing exercises, and your joints will bear the stress from this extra weight. Proper technique is what will prevent the risk of injuries, so please pay particular attention to the directions for each exercise. To further eliminate the risk of injury, all of the exercises outlined for your legs will be performed on machines that can be found at almost every athletic facility. These machines are designed to reduce stress on your joints, and because their working parts are primarily cables, pulleys and weight, there is little or no fear of the actual weight causing injury or harm.

The walking lunge is arguably one of the finest exercises for creating shape from the waist down. You will really feel this exercise in the buttocks and in the thighs. This exercise is designed to be an effective warm-up for all the muscles in the legs. Do it outdoors, in a relatively long hallway, on the basketball floor, or on an empty racquetball court. The walking lunge can be performed to accommodate any level of fitness, with only modest alterations.

Get Ready

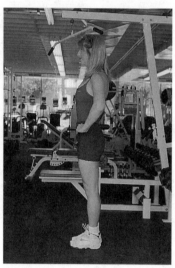

Beginners: With your legs a comfortable distance apart, stand with your hands on your hips.

Advanced: With your legs a comfortable distance apart, stand with a dumbbell in each hand. Allow your arms to be fully extended, and your hands to hang down next to your thighs. They will remain in this position throughout the exercise. The more advanced you become, the greater the weight.

Very Advanced: Put on your weight vest. Stand with your legs a comfortable distance apart, and place your hands on your hips.

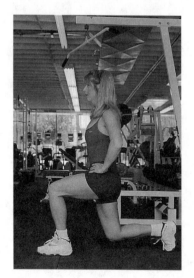

The Exercise

From the standing position, inhale and step forward with your left leg, landing on your heel. With your left foot flat against the ground, bend your right knee until it is at a 90° angle. Keep the torso straight and allow the right heel to raise as you come down and almost touch the ground with your left knee, and hold for one count. Your legs should now be in the shape of a box. Exhale and come up, pressing through the left heel. When your legs are fully extended, bring the feet together and repeat with your right leg. Perform the prescribed number of paces (at least 20), and stretch after each set.

Stretch

Standing with your feet together, bring your left heel toward your buttocks. If you need to, you may certainly use your right hand to balance or brace yourself against something sturdy. Hold your left ankle with your left hand, bringing the heel closer and closer toward the buttocks. Continue stretching for 30 seconds. Repeat on the right side.

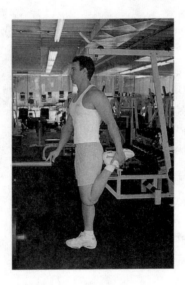

This is one of the most perfect exercises for developing, toning, and working the front of the thigh. Even if your legs are the same size or you have developed the legs to be the same exact size, you should perform this exercise one leg at a time, at least once a week, so that a more dominant (and bigger) leg does not develop.

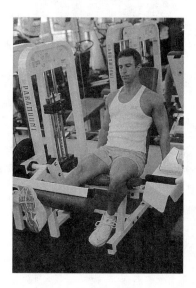

Get Ready

For this exercise your focus is as pointed to the "negative" movement as much as it is concerned with moving the weight. When you come down at the bottom of this movement, the weight plates can touch, but under no circumstances should there be any slapping or banging of metal. To get the most out of the leg extension, do not simply throw the weight up with your leg, but drive the weight up, hold at the top of the movement, and ease the weight back down slowly. This will have great effects in terms of the eventual shape of your leg.

Sit down on the leg extension machine, with your back long against the chair, and make certain that you do not rock while you perform this exercise. Place your hands on the grips provided to you, or grasp the seat of the chair. Place both feet behind the pad provided to you on this machine. Do not point your toes, rather flex the foot by bringing the toes up.

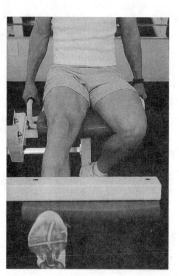

The Exercise

Begin with the right leg. Exhale and drive the weight up, until your leg is fully extended. Hold the weight at this position for one count, inhale and release the leg back down slowly on a count of three-two-one. Hold at the bottom of the movement as you finish your inhalation. Exhale and repeat the prescribed number of repetitions. Perform the same number of repetitions with your left leg to complete the set. Stretch after each set.

Stretch

Stand up straight, and with your knees close together, extend one of your arms, and use your right arm to brace yourself on something that won't move. (Try not to put your hand on another machine somebody else is using.) Bring your left heel toward your buttocks. Grasp your left ankle with the left hand and bring the heel as close to the buttocks as you comfortably can. Hold this stretch for thirty seconds, then repeat on your right side.

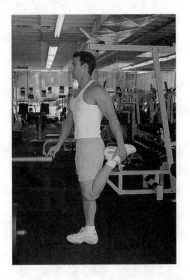

LEG CURLS

Leg curls are performed on machines which facilitate either a sitting or prone position and are designed to work the back of the thigh. Not only is this muscle vital in terms of athletic performance but it is a very large muscle, which is capable of almost infinite growth in terms of muscle density. The more defined and larger this muscle becomes, the more balanced and attractive the aesthetic appearance of your legs.

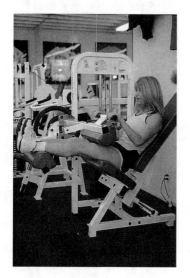

SEATED LEG CURL

Get Ready

This exercise is performed on a machine that is built around a chair. There is a padded cushion at the back of the ankles and often a bar that comes down over your lap, much like rides at the amusement park. In the seated position, the basic motion of this exercise is to drive the lower part of your legs back as far as the machine allows. Weights are selected to provide resistance for the movement. After you are seated in the chair, please adjust the height and depth of the chair so that the moving hinge is exactly even with your knee.

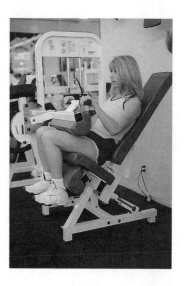

The Exercise

After making the proper adjustments, sit down in the chair and lower the bar to keep your thighs in place. Flex your foot by raising the toes higher than your heel. This exercise should be performed one leg at a time until muscular balance has been achieved. Exhale and drive the right heel back as far as possible. Hold for one count. Inhale and slowly release your leg back to the starting position on a count of three-two-one, without letting the weight plates touch the stack. Hold this position for one count. Repeat for the prescribed number of repetitions, and then perform the exact same number of repetitions with the left leg. Stretch after each set.

Get Ready

As opposed to sitting, this exercise is performed lying face down on a flat bench. The basic movement for this exercise is to bring your heels to your buttocks. There is an extension on the bench with two cylindrical-shaped cushions. When lying on your stomach, these cushions should be just above the back of your ankles. Often there are handgrips or a place to rest your forearms. If not, simply grip the corners of

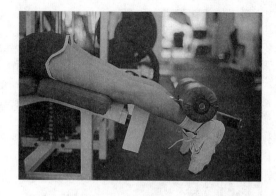

the bench nearest your head. Again, the moving hinge of this machine should be exactly even with your knee. Don't let the cushion roll up your calf.

The Exercise

This exercise should be performed one leg at a time until muscular balance has been achieved. In the prone position, exhale and drive your right heel to your buttocks. When you get as close as you can, raise the entire thigh one or two inches above the bench, intensifying the flex in the back of the

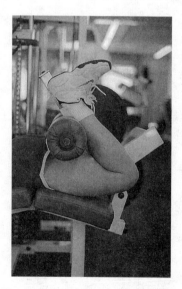

thigh. Hold this position for one count. Inhale and release your thigh back down to the bench and lower your leg back to the starting position on a count of three-two-one, without letting the weights touch the stack. Repeat for the prescribed number of repetitions, then perform the same number of repetitions with your left leg. Stretch after each set.

Stretch for Both Leg Curls

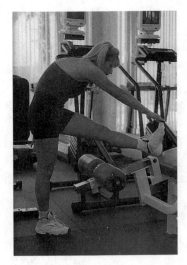

Stand up and find a stable object that is about the same height as your waist. Place your right heel on top on the object and flex your foot by bringing the toes back toward you. With your torso square to the right leg, bring the torso down toward your right thigh and try to grasp your foot with both hands. With every exhalation gradually lower the torso and deepen the stretch without bouncing. You should feel this stretch from your heel through your buttock along the length of your hamstring. Continue to stretch for at least 30 seconds, then repeat on your left leg.

INNER THIGH AND OUTER THIGH

These two exercises are designed to work the muscles of the inner and outer thigh. There are very few activities that we perform during our day to hit these muscles. As a consequence, these particular areas often lack tone and definition. Both of these exercises are tremendously important in working these hard-to-reach areas.

INNER THIGH

Get Ready

This exercise is performed on the adductor machine. Make certain that the chair on this machine is positioned at the right height, making the pad for your legs exactly even with your knees. The basic motion of this exercise is to bring your knees together.

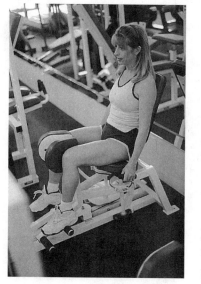

The Exercise

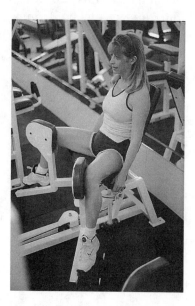

Sit in the chair and spread your legs as wide as you comfortably can until the machine locks into the widest possible setting. Exhale and bring your knees together. Hold for one count as you finish your exhalation. Inhale and slowly come back to your starting position on a count of three-two-one. Repeat for the prescribed number of repetitions. Stretch after each set.

Stretch

With your legs still spread wide in the starting position, lean over and grasp the machine on either side with both of your hands. Keep your back straight, and lower your torso between your legs without bouncing. Allow yourself to go lower and lower with each exhalation. Continue stretching for at least 30 seconds.

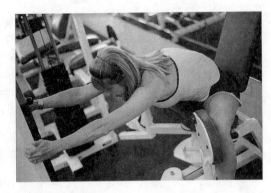

OUTER THIGH

Get Ready

This exercise is performed on the abductor machine. Again, make certain that the chair is positioned in such a way to position your knees against the pad. Lean forward until your torso is just above your thighs, and hold onto either side of the machine with each hand. (Be careful that your hands are not in the way of the weight plates or on the track that allows the weights to move.)

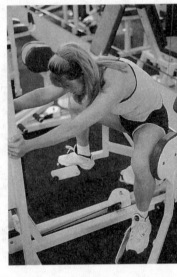

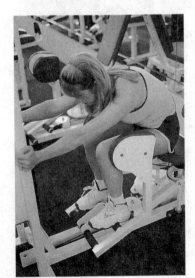

The Exercise

Exhale and drive the knees out as wide as you can. Hold this position for one count, as you finish your exhalation. Inhale, and slowly bring the knees back to your starting position on a count of three-two-one. Repeat for the prescribed number of repetitions. Stretch after each set.

Stretch

Lean back and sit straight up in the chair. Bring your right leg up and over the left, so the back of the right knee is lying on top of your left knee. Place your left hand on your right knee and gently pull it toward your left shoulder. Continue this stretch for 30 seconds. Repeat this stretch for the left leg.

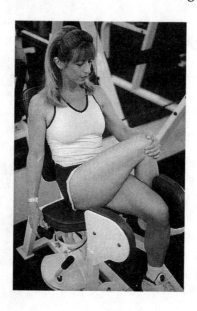

CALF RAISE

The calf muscles can be worked from either a standing position or on the leg press machine. Although these muscles do get frequent use, most people would like better definition in these muscles. The calf raise is designed to heighten definition and to create a perfect finish for the leg in terms of aesthetic appearance.

STANDING CALF RAISE

Get Ready

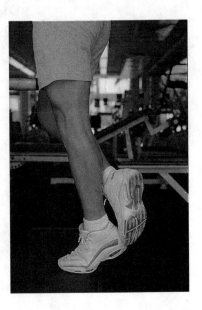

Find a raised object, such as a step used for aerobics, a platform without a lip, or even a bench. Stand on top of the object in such a way that your heels are unimpeded. Move back so that the only contact between your foot and the object you are standing on are the ball of your foot and your toes. Allow the heels to lower as far as possible, and feel the stretch through the back of your calves. Place the top of your right foot just above the heel of your left foot. If you need to hold onto something for balance, you may certainly do so, but do not support your weight with that object.

The Exercise

Allow your left heel to sink as far as it possibly can. Exhale and drive up with your left foot until you are standing, tippy-toed, on the ball of your left foot. Inhale and lower yourself down on a count of three-two-one as your heel reaches toward the floor. Hold at the bottom for one count and feel the stretch through the back of your calf as you finish your exhalation. Exhale and repeat the movement for the prescribed number of repetitions.

Stretch

Stretch after each set by remaining in the heel-down position for at least 30 seconds. Repeat on the other side.

Get Ready

The seated calf raise is performed on the leg press machine. Sit down in the chair that this machine provides. Place your feet on the sled, unlock the latch holding the sled in place, and extend your legs fully. Adjust your feet so that the balls of your feet are just above the lower edge of the sled. Allow your toes to come back toward you as far as possible and feel the stretch through the back of your calves.

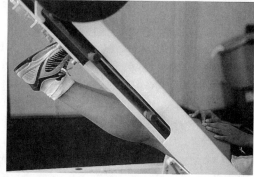

The Exercise

Exhale and drive up until the balls of your feet and the toes are the only things holding the sled up. Inhale and lower your toes down toward you on a count of three-two-one as your heel reaches away from you as far as possible. Hold this position for one count and feel the stretch through the back of your calf as you finish your exhalation. Exhale and repeat the movement for the prescribed number of repetitions.

Stretch

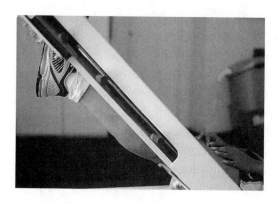

Stretch after each set by remaining in the starting position for at least 30 seconds. Repeat on the left side.

BUTT KICKS

Designed specifically to work the gluteus maximus, or butt muscles, this exercise will strengthen, shape, and tone all areas of your backside.

Get Ready

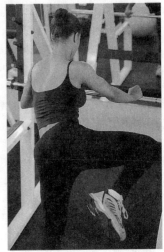

Find a solid object that is about chest high and can support your weight. In the picture you can see that we have used a barbell on the squat rack, but you could easily use a banister or the handrail of any staircase landing. Stand away from the bar, place both hands slightly wider than shoulder-width apart, and lean forward so that your torso is at a 45° angle with the floor. Bring your right knee and right heel up to the side until they are parallel to the floor, then bring your heel toward your buttocks until your leg is at a 90° angle.

The Exercise

Exhale and push through your heel, until your leg is completely straight and there is a line from your heel to your head. Inhale and bring your heel to your buttocks, coming back to your starting position on a count of three-two-one. Hold and repeat the prescribed number of repetitions, then repeat on your left side.

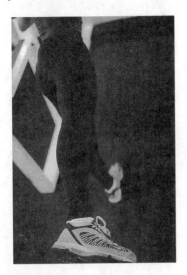

Stretch

Stand up tall with your arms at your sides. Drop your chin to your chest. Let the weight of your head pull you down vertebra by vertebra. Allow your arms to hang down so that your fingers point toward your toes. Touch your toes, or come as close as your hamstrings will allow you to. If you can easily touch your toes, try to touch the palms of your hands against the floor. If you are especially limber, cross your arms and try to touch your elbows to the floor. Above all, keep the motion constant and avoid bouncing. Maintain this continuous stretch, and try to deepen it for at least 30 seconds.

HOT POINT FITNESS

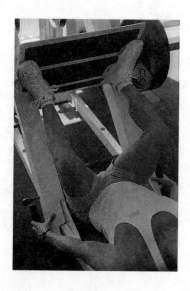

This exercise is designed to work the entire leg. Maximizing this exercise to hit all the leg muscles requires proper foot position and impeccable technique. The most important factor to be concerned about is eliminating the possibility of knee injuries. The knee joint will have considerable stress placed upon it throughout this exercise, and to reduce any associated risk, proper foot placement is essential.

Get Ready

Your feet should be placed shoulder-width apart on the plate directly in front of you, and they should be pointed out slightly. This helps to ensure that you are pushing the weight

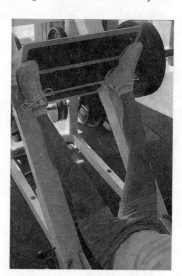

with and through your heels. When the leg is fully extended there will be a straight line from your heels to your buttocks. **DO NOT** push with your toes. This dramatically increases the strain on your knee joints, and if you perform this exercise pushing with your toes, you will not get the full benefit of the exercise and also risk painful injuries.

Sit down on the seat of the leg press machine. Feel your lower back against the chair, and keep the back supported in this way throughout the exercise.

The Exercise

Exhale and drive the weight up until the legs are fully extended. **Do not lock your knees.** Hold in this position for one count. Inhale and slowly release the knees toward your chest on a count of three-two-one. Bring the weight down until your buttocks are just about to come up off the seat. Hold this position for one count as you finish your inhalation. Exhale and repeat the prescribed number of repetitions.

Create Muscle Strength at a Deeper Level . . . Quickly

Stretch

Stand up tall with your arms at your sides. Drop your chin to your chest. Let the weight of your head pull you down vertebra by vertebra. Allow your arms to hang down so that your fingers point toward your toes. Touch your toes, or come as close as your hamstrings will allow you to. If you can easily touch your toes, try to touch the palms of your hands against the floor. If you are especially limber, cross your arms, and try to touch your elbows to the floor. Above all, keep the motion constant, and avoid bouncing. Maintain this continuous stretch, and try to deepen it for at least 30 seconds.

THE SQUAT

The squat is designed to work each and every muscle from the waist down and is the king of all leg exercises. This exercise is physically taxing and is one of the most aerobically demanding resistance-training exercises ever devised. Because the squat is one of the most difficult exercises to perform correctly, I will introduce this exercise slowly into your workouts and provide three stages to safely master the perfect technique. All stages work equally well for the leg muscles. But as you become more advanced, in terms of your technique, you will gradually add weight to continue benefiting from the exercise.

SQUAT #1

Get Ready

No matter at what level you are currently exercising, I strongly suggest that you begin at this stage. This exercise is designed to instill the perfect and ideal squat technique.

Find a bench or chair. When seated, your thighs should not be any lower than parallel to the floor. Stand with your back to the bench or chair and place your arms in the "I Dream of Genie" pose. Your feet should be turned out slightly and planted firmly on the floor, slightly wider than shoulder-width apart.

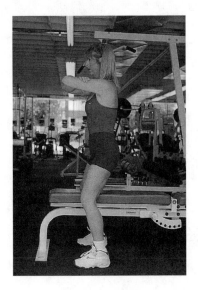

The Exercise

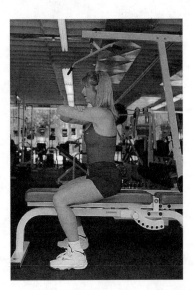

Keeping your head and spine in alignment, inhale, bend your knees, and allow your butt to go back as if you were going to sit on the bench or chair on a count of three-two-one. Just as you begin to make contact

Create Muscle Strength at a Deeper Level . . . Quickly

with the bench or chair, hold for one count then exhale and drive up through the heels, until you return to a standing position. Repeat for the prescribed number of repetitions. Stretch after each set.

Stretch for All Squat Exercises

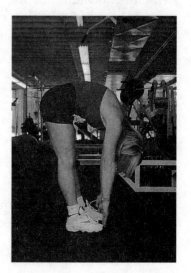

Stand up tall with your arms at your sides. Drop your chin to your chest. Let the weight of your head pull you down vertebra by vertebra. Allow your arms to hang down so that your fingers are going toward your toes. Touch your toes, or come as close as your hamstrings will allow you to. If you can easily touch your toes, try to touch the palms of your hands against the floor. If you are especially limber, cross your arms and try to touch your elbows to the floor. Above all, keep the motion constant and avoid bouncing. Maintain this continuous stretch, and try to deepen it for at least 30 seconds.

Get Ready

With a dumbbell in each hand, and your arms hanging at your sides, stand with your back to a bench or chair of appropriate height. Your feet should be turned out slightly and planted firmly on the floor, slightly wider than shoulder-width apart.

The Exercise

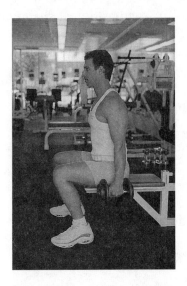

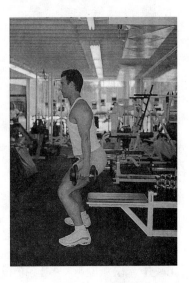

Keeping your head and spine in alignment, inhale, bend your knees, and allow your butt to go back as if you were going to sit on the bench or chair on a count of three-two-one. Just as the buttocks begin to make contact, hold for one count, then exhale and drive up through the heels, extending the legs until you return to a standing position. Repeat for the prescribed number of repetitions. Stretch after each set.

This exercise is an extremely advanced one, and executing the squat with perfect technique is essential. The most important factor is positioning. This exercise is to be performed with a bar and a squat rack. You should begin by using the bar only. It weighs approximately 45 pounds. Gradually increase the weight over an extended period of time. I prefer to use a pad in the center of the bar, as it eases the strain and any irritation of the bar against the bones.

Get Ready

With the bar on the rack, come up from under the bar until your shoulder blades make contact. Let the bar meet the top of your shoulder blades below the bottom

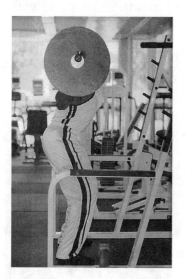

of your neck. Place your hands on the bar, taking a fairly wide grip. Usually the area of the bar that accommodates your hands has a rough finish to facilitate a better grip. The center of this grip is marked with either a smooth surface, an indentation, or a raised ring. Place the middle finger of each hand on this center-point. With your legs positioned slightly wider than shoulder-width apart, bend your knees and bring your body directly under the bar. Straighten your legs and lift the bar off the squat rack. Take a few steps backward until you have cleared the rack and stand up tall, facing the mirror. Make any necessary adjustments, positioning yourself in the proper starting position.

The Exercise

Facing the mirror, your feet should be turned out slightly and planted firmly on the floor, slightly wider than shoulder-width apart. Keeping your head and spine in alignment, inhale, bend your knees, and allow your butt to go back as if you were going to sit on an imaginary bench on a count of three-two-one. It is very important that you be looking straight ahead with your spine in a straight line and your neck long and straight. Continue to bend the knees, and jut out the buttocks until your legs are at a 90° angle. Hold this position for one count. Exhale and drive up through the heels, extending the legs until you return to a standing position. Repeat for the prescribed number of repetitions. Stretch after each set.

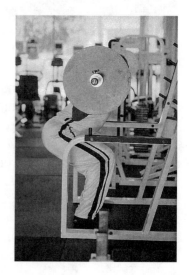

YOUR ABDOMINAL MUSCLES

The abdominal muscles are grouped in blocks that form a checkerboard pattern across the middle of your body. For your workout purposes, the abdominal muscles will be separated into three areas: the upper, middle, and lower abdominal muscles.

The basic strategy here is to perform one exercise for the top, one exercise for the middle, and one exercise for the bottom of the abdominal muscles. Like aerobic activity, you may do abdominal exercises as many as six times per week. As with any form of exercise, you must rest at least one day per week to let the body rest and heal itself.

The abdominals develop by contracting the muscles, and does not depend on stretching to create an elongated look. Getting your stomach to look the way you want it to look, however, does not necessarily mean that you have to do 20,000 sit-ups a day. Abdominal exercises only develop the musculature under the skin. Getting the washboard look, or the 6-pack, is truly a function of diet and aerobics. I promise that you already have a six-pack. The problem is that there is fat on top of it, and because of the fat under the skin, you cannot see this muscular separation. To develop these particular muscles, you will work the lower portion more intensely. The lower portion of the abdominal wall is almost always the most underdeveloped musculature in the body. By paying particular attention to these muscles, you create a foundation to build upon. In addition, the lower abdominal exercises will also help to develop the middle and upper portions of this region.

Muscular development throughout the abdominal region not only accentuates and heightens appearance but it is also beneficial to your overall health. As the abdominal region supports the body, strengthening this area can offset or prevent back problems, improve our posture, and in doing so, enhance circulation. If you have ever had back pain, you know that there is no pain that can compare to it. The abdominal muscles are precisely what keeps the spine in alignment, and if you do have back pain, it may be exactly this form of exercise that can bring some needed relief. As a preventative measure against future back problems, there is nothing that can equal a solid abdominal exercise routine performed regularly.

As you become more advanced and feel the need to do more of these exercises than is recommended in your workouts, I strongly suggest that you begin to add weights. This can be accomplished quite easily. For any of the following exercises that require you to lift your legs, simply put on a pair of ankle weights. For any of the following exercises which call for you to raise your torso, you may perform the exercise either by holding a weight plate to your chest with both arms, or by holding the weight plate behind your head with both hands.

THE CRUNCH

The "crunch" is just an improvement over the most basic form of sit-up. The movement is to bring your elbows to your knees. The key to getting the most abdominal work is to get the great majority of your hip off the ground as you fold your body. It is a fantastic overall abdominal muscle exercise and is even great for those of you with back problems. To minimize neck injuries, do not pull your head up with your hands; let the stomach muscles do the work of the crunch instead. The point is to contract the abdominal muscles, and not to give them any rest during the exercise. To keep the contraction going throughout the exercise, perform these as slowly as possible.

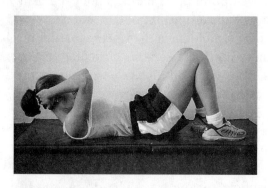

Get Ready

Either place your hands beneath your head, or place them on the opposite shoulder.

Begin the exercise with your head and feet on the mat.

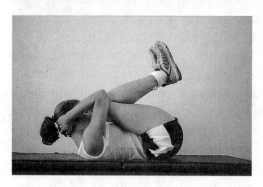

The Exercise

Bring your chin to your chest. Exhale as you bring your knees towards your elbows. Pull your belly button in toward your spine. Hold at the top of the crunch as you finish the exhalation. Inhale as you slowly release the contraction. When you feel the point at which you lose the contraction, stop, exhale, and slowly bring the knees towards the elbows again.

Get Ready

This sit-up is performed on the Roman Chair. For this particular exercise, you should situate yourself in the chair so that your ankles are behind the cushion for your feet and your buttocks are resting against the back cushions. You may perform this exercise with your arms crossed across your chest and your hands on the opposite shoulders, or in the "I Dream of Genie" position, or by holding a weight plate to your chest.

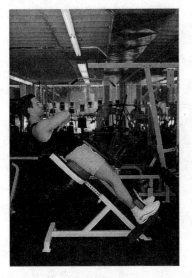

The Exercise

Lean back so that you are actually standing in the machine held in place by the ankle pads. Make your body as straight as possible in this inclined position. Make a note of the position and do not go any further back than you are at this time, as this will cause undue strain on your lower back. Pull your belly button toward your spine. Exhale and, keeping the spine and head straight, slowly bring your torso forward on a count of one-two-three, as far as you can until you reach the point when you just begin to lose tension in the abdominal muscles. Hold in this position for one count. Inhale and slowly release the torso back to the starting position on a count of four-three-two-one. The negative movement in this exercise is critical and will work the abdominal muscles very hard. Perform the prescribed number of repetitions.

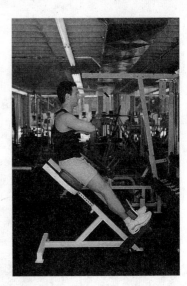

HAND CRUNCH

The "hand crunch" is just a variation of the previous crunch and is designed for those with a bad back or a bad neck. The movement is quite similar. You will be folding and unfolding the body using your abdominal muscles. The only difference is hand and arm placement. Again, the point of this exercise is to create a constant contraction for the abdominal muscles. The point at which you begin to lose the contraction marks the limitations to your range of motion.

Get Ready

Place your hands, palms down, underneath your buttocks. Make a diamond shape out of your index fingers and thumbs. Rest your tailbone over the diamond. Begin this exercise with your head and feet on the ground.

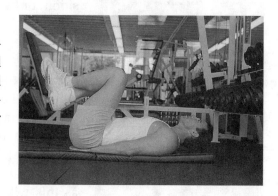

The Exercise

With your head and shoulders firmly planted, pull your belly button toward your spine and exhale as you raise your legs. Lift your hips off the ground as your knees bend, and slowly bring your knees into (or as close as you can to) your chest. Hold your position at the end of this movement and finish your exhalation. (As you become more advanced, you may add ankle weights.) Inhale as you slowly unfold. When you feel the point at which you just begin to lose the contraction, stop, exhale, and repeat the movement.

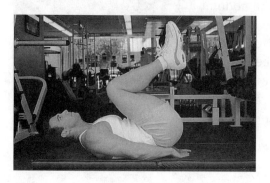
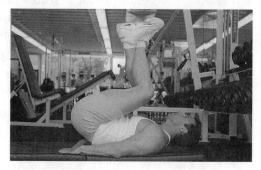

This exercise is designed to work the whole abdominal region. Let the abdominal muscles do the work of lifting the torso, and you will get the most out of this exercise. The point of this exercise is to keep the shoulders and as much of the buttocks as you can off the ground to ensure constant abdominal contraction.

Get Ready

Lie on your back with your legs straight up in the air, so that you are positioned at a 90° angle or "L" shape. Cross your ankles, bend your knees, and let your feet drop about three inches. Either place your hands beneath your head or cross your arms "mummy-style" over your chest and place your hands on the opposite shoulder.

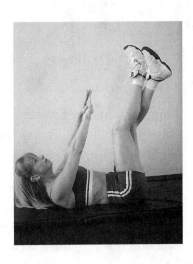

The Exercise

Bring your knees towards your head so your buttocks come off the ground. Pull your belly button in toward your spine. Exhale as you slowly bring your torso towards your knees. Hold your position at the top of the movement as you finish your exhalation. Inhale as you slowly release your torso towards the ground. At the point at which you begin to lose the abdominal contraction, exhale and repeat the motion.

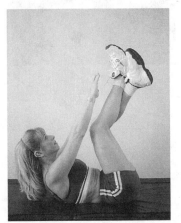

BUTT LIFT

This exercise is an excellent choice for working the lower abdominal muscles. Similar in some ways to the toe touch, this exercise is perhaps the finest lower abdominal exercise in existence.

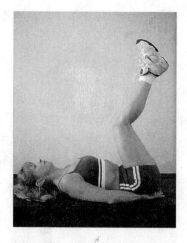

Get Ready

To begin this exercise, lie flat on your back with your arms to your sides, palms flat on the mat under your hips with your fingers spread.

The Exercise

Cross your ankles. Bring your knees up toward your face. Extend the lower legs straight up until the knees are only slightly bent. Using your hands for support, exhale, pull your belly button in, and use your lower abdominal muscles to drive your heels up toward the ceiling. Continue to lift up until the buttocks are completely off the mat. Hold for one count in the up position as you finish your exhalation. Inhale and come down slowly. Exhale and repeat for the prescribed number of repetitions.

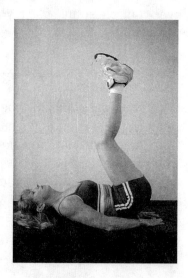

This exercise is designed to work the abdominal musculature diagonally, to fully develop all four corners of the muscle group. This exercise is designed to hit every block in your checkerboard. To get the most out of this exercise, keep your torso in a raised and fixed position. While pumping the legs as if you were on a bicycle, touch your elbow to the opposite knee on every pump of your legs. The point is not to do this exercise slowly, but to keep the contraction as you reach your elbows as far as you can to the left and to the right.[1]

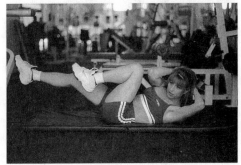

Get Ready

Lie flat on your back with the backs of your legs and your head resting against the ground. Interlock your fingers, and place your hands beneath your head. Keeping the legs straight, lift your feet 8 inches above the floor.

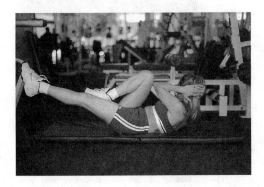

The Exercise

Bend your left knee and bring it towards your chest as the shoulders and upper torso come up off the ground. Touch your right elbow to your left knee. Keeping the torso in the same position, release the left leg back to the starting position and touch your left elbow to your right knee.

---

[1]If you have neck or back problems, you may want to avoid this particular exercise.

THE PENGUIN

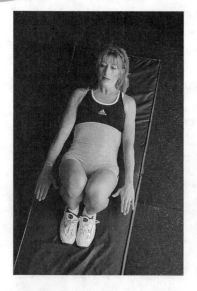

This exercise is designed to create strength and definition along the edges of the abdominal musculature and is a fantastic exercise for the oblique muscles.

The point is to keep your shoulders and torso off the ground for the entire exercise.

Get Ready

Lie flat on your back with your arms along your sides, palms against the floor. Bend your knees and bring your feet as close as you can to your buttocks. Place your feet flat on the ground so your knees are pointed toward the ceiling.

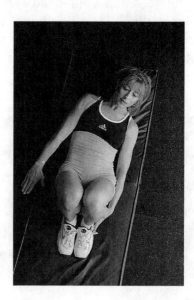

The Exercise

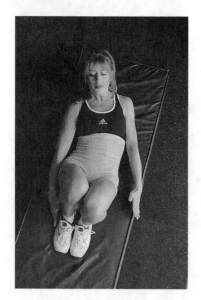

Tuck your chin into your chest, lifting your head, shoulders, and upper torso off the ground. Touch your right heel with your right hand. Touch your left heel with your left hand. Alternate between the right and the left quickly, and you will soon discover how this exercise was named.

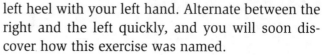

This exercise is designed to work the blocks of abdominal muscles diagonally across the stomach and will effectively reach all the areas of this muscle group.

Get Ready

Lie flat on your back with the soles of your feet against the mat and your knees pointed toward the ceiling. Cross your legs, placing the outside of your right ankle on top of your left knee. The crossed leg remains stationary throughout the exercise.

The Exercise

Pull your belly button in toward your spine. Exhale and try to touch your left elbow to your right knee, bringing the shoulder blades and upper back off the mat. Inhale and come down without letting your shoulderblades rest against the mat. Exhale and repeat for the prescribed number of repetitions. Repeat on the other side.

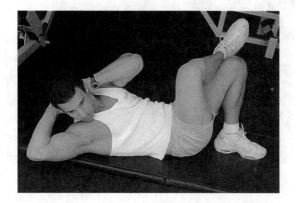

SIDE CRUNCH AND
ROMAN CHAIR SIDE CRUNCH

These two exercises are very similar in that they are designed to specifically target the oblique muscles. Whenever you see the "SIDE CRUNCH" prescribed in your daily workout, you may choose either of these exercises.

SIDE CRUNCH

The basic movement for this exercise is exactly like a sit-up. You are bringing your head, shoulders, and upper back off the mat as you bring your torso straight up.

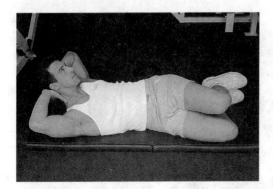

Get Ready

Lie on the mat with your feet flat and your knees pointed toward the ceiling. Drop both of your knees to the right side, without losing contact between your back and the mat. Interlock your fingers and place your hands behind your head.

The Exercise

Exhale and bring the torso straight up as if you were performing a sit-up, lifting as high as you possibly can. Inhale and come down slowly on a count of three-two-one. Without letting your shoulder blades rest against the mat, exhale and repeat for the prescribed number of repetitions. Perform the exact same number of repetitions with your knees pointed to your left.

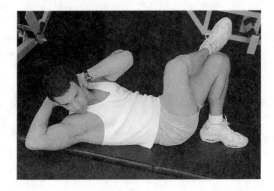

This is definitely the more advanced of the two exercises.

Get Ready

Situate yourself in the Roman chair so that your right hip is pressed against the back cushion and your left ankle is pressed against the foot cushion. Your right foot is planted against the brace of the footrest as if you were taking a walking stride with your legs. Interlock your fingers and place them behind your head.

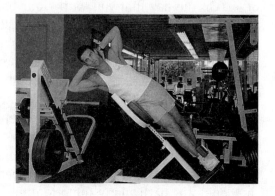

The Exercise

Inhale and drop the right elbow toward the floor on a count of four-three-two-one. Hold in this position a count of three to feel the stretch. Exhale and come back to your starting position. Repeat for the prescribed number of repetitions.

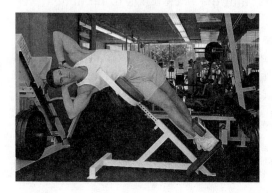

YOUR BACK

The back is made up of several muscles and muscle groups that enable you to lift, pull, bend, and twist. Working all of these muscle groups requires separate and distinct exercises, because they in large part operate independently from one another. On the day that you work your back you will perform several exercises to aid in the development of your back muscles.

Most people, even professional bodybuilders, have a problem developing the muscles in the back. Usually, the main problem is that they are working their arms more than their back muscles. If you fail to focus on this important muscle group, you will not only fail to develop a balanced aesthetic look but you may also risk depriving yourself of an important weapon to combat future back-related problems. Because all of us have a tendency to use our arm muscles more than those located on the back when we pull an object, we lack the capacity to actually contract these important muscles. While performing the exercises in this section of the book, it is particularly important to contract these muscles as much as possible. This contraction will not only enable development much more rapidly but you will grow to depend on these muscles more heavily in your everyday life. You will consequently lower the risk of injuring your back.

Because the back muscles are not a priority for most people, this muscle group tends to be overlooked. Men have a tendency to want a developed bicep. And you can see, even in professional bodybuilders, that the back tends to be underdeveloped. In essence, if you do not see it, you are not that concerned about it. Women however, tend to pay attention to this area much more frequently. Backless dresses and evening gowns often reveal this area, and the greater the muscular definition in this area, the more flattering the dress. As men and women have different needs and desires in terms of muscular development, you will generally see that difference reflected in the number of repetitions required for each exercise in your workout.

Specifically because most of us are not used to flexing the back muscles, it is important to begin the process of flexing as part of this exercise. This exercise is designed to strengthen and define your lateral muscles. Developing these muscles can make your waistline look slimmer and give your back an attractive aesthetic. Just to reiterate, when you are finished with each set, you should feel this more in your back than in your arms. To accomplish this, be strict about your technique.

Get Ready

This exercise is performed on the lat pull-down machine. Place your hands on the bar just slightly wider than shoulder-width apart. While holding onto the bar, sit down on the attached stool. Place your feet on the floor so that your knees are bent and in a comfortable and relaxed position.

You should begin to feel an effective stretch as the weight lifts your arms higher. This exercise begins by flexing your back muscles. Before attempting this exercise for the first time, experience this flex by engaging the muscles of the shoulder blades. While you are in this position, squeeze your shoulder blades together. Keep squeezing and come as close as you can to having the shoulder blades touch. From now on I will refer to this as "engaging the shoulder blades."

The Exercise

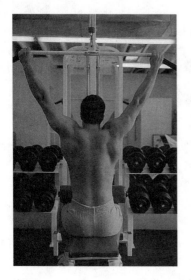

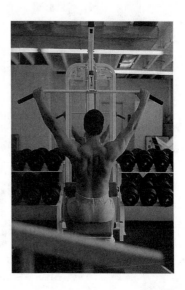

This exercise is performed using a count of six. On count one engage the shoulder blades by flexing the back, or squeezing the shoulder blades together. Count two is an explosive motion bringing the bar to the middle of your chest. Hold this position on count three and main-

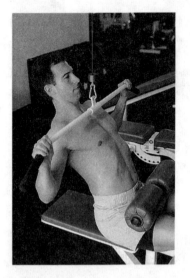

tain the flex of your back muscles. On a count of four – five – six, let the bar go up slowly. At the count of six, release the flex and enjoy the full stretch.

Stretch

Find a pole that is solid enough to support your weight. Place your feet on either side of the base of that pole. Interlock your fingers around the pole and place your hands above your head. Let the weight of your buttocks and torso fall away from the pole and allow your body to form the shape of an archer's bow. Feel the stretch between your shoulder blades and along the length of your back. Perform this stretch for 40 seconds after each set.

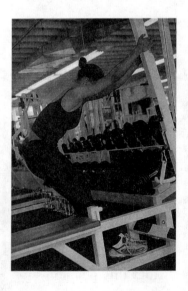

This exercise is designed to work the shoulder blades and the middle portion of your back. Like the lat pull down, special attention is given to engaging the shoulder blades. Flexing the muscles in your back is an integral part of the exercise. This is not a workout for your arms. The point is to depend more on the muscles of your back.

Get Ready

The seated row is performed on the seated row machine, or can be performed on the cable machine seated on the ground. The hand grips for this exercise should be a butterfly-shape, or two D-shaped hand grips. Your knees should be bent and raised slightly, as if you were in a rowing scull or on the rowing machine. Unlike rowing, your legs will remain in this position and will not straighten during the exercise.

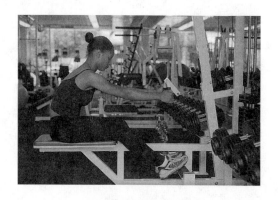

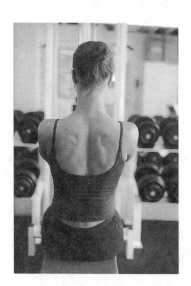

The Exercise

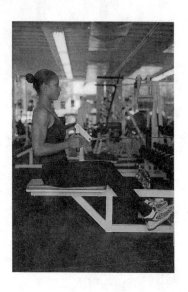

Exhale as you engage the shoulder blades. Pull the bar below your rib cage. Hold for a one count. Inhale on a count of three-two-one, easing the weight back toward your starting position until your arms are fully extended. Release the flex in your back muscles and let the weight pull your torso forward until you are enjoying a nice stretch along your back. Exhale and repeat for the prescribed number of repetitions.

Stretch after each set using the example on page 72.

The One Arm Row is an excellent exercise to develop your back and to promote a muscular balance between your right and left side. Like the lat pull down and seated row, particular attention should be paid to engaging the shoulder blades.

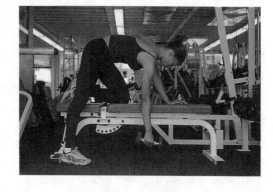

Get Ready

This exercise is performed using one dumbbell. Using a flat bench, plant your left knee and left palm flat on the bench to stabilize yourself. Your back should be flat, and your head should be in alignment with your spine so you are looking at the top of the bench. Extend your right hand and grip the dumbbell. Feel the weight gently stretch the muscles along your right shoulder blade. Keeping your right arm straight and long, engage the right shoulder blade.

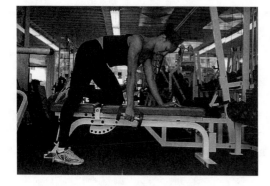

The Exercise

Exhale and, with an explosive motion, bring the right elbow up and above your back until it is pointed straight at the ceiling. The motion is like sawing a piece of wood. Hold this position for one count. Inhale and lower your fist

toward the floor on a count of three-two-one. Feel the stretch through your back and shoulder as you finish your inhalation. Repeat the prescribed number of repetitions, and repeat the same exact number on your left side. Remember to work to the weak side. Stretch after each set using the back stretch described for the previous exercise.

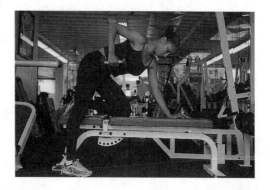

THE HYPER-EXTENSION

The hyper-extension is one of the most fantastic exercises for the lower back. This exercise will do a great deal to improve your posture and addresses longevity issues effectively. It is a fantastic exercise for those with back problems, who have weakness in their lower backs, and for those who have suffered injury to that area of the body. If you have not had an injury to this area, performing this exercise could further prevent having one. For this reason alone, the hyper-extension is one of the finest preventative exercises.[2]

There are two ways to perform this exercise. For my clients who are either beginning elderly or rehabilitating from a lower back injury, I recommend performing this exercise with the aid of a therapy ball. For people that do not have injury concerns, this exercise can be performed on the hyper-extension machine. In both exercises, the movement for this exercise is not an explosive one. The point of this exercise is to maintain a slow and even pace. The motion should be fluid, and you should, above all, avoid any jerking movements.

---

[2]As you become more advanced, you can begin adding weight for this exercise. Simply use both arms to hold a weight plate to your chest, and complete the exercise as described above.

DIRECTION 1 – FOR THOSE WITH LOWER BACK CONCERNS

Get Ready

With the therapy ball on the floor, kneel beside it and place your tummy on the ball. Bring your arms over the ball, and roll forward slowly until your body is draped over the ball. Bring your knees up off the ground, and place the soles of your feet against the wall. Stay there for several moments, experimenting with the position that best elongates the spine. Feel the wonderful stretch through the length of your back. Perform this stretch for two minutes before and after this exercise.

The Exercise

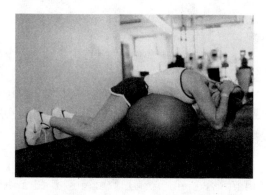

Either put your hands behind your head, or place your hands on the opposite elbow in the "I Dream of Genie" position, depending on what is more comfortable for you. Keeping your head in alignment with your torso, and your face pointed toward the floor, inhale and slowly bring your torso up on a count of four – three – two – one, your knees and head are in a straight line. Hold the torso in this position for one count as you finish your inhalation. Exhale and slowly release your body down on a

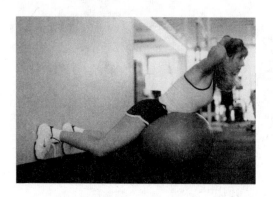

count of three – two – one, until you are draped over the ball in your starting position. Repeat as directed. Remember to stretch for at least one minute between sets, and two minutes when you are finished with the prescribed number of sets.

DIRECTION 2

Get Ready

Stand on the hyper-extension machine with your pelvis facing the pad and the back of your ankles against the footrest. Depending on what is more comfortable, either interlock your fingers and place your hands behind your head or cross your

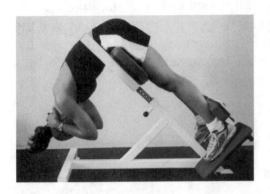

arms over your chest, mummy style, placing your hands on the opposite shoulders.

The Exercise

With your torso erect and your spine straight, exhale and slowly let the weight of your arms pull you toward the floor on a count of three–two–one, hold for one count. Inhale and slowly bring your torso up on a count of three–two–one, until your spine is straight and your head is aligned with your feet. Hold this position for one count. Exhale and repeat.

   As you become more advanced, you can begin adding weight for this exercise. Simply use both arms to hold a weight plate to your chest, and complete the exercise as described above.

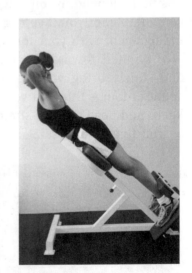

Stretch

Standing upright with your feet together, let your head fall forward and let your chin touch your chest. Let the weight of your head and shoulders slowly pull your head toward the floor. Come as close as you can to touching your toes and hold for 30 seconds. If you are very limber, cross your arms and see if you can touch your elbows to the floor. Slowly come back up, stacking one vertebra on top of another. Your head is the last thing that stacks on top of the spine.

The shrugs are an ideal exercise to work the trapezius muscles, or "traps" as they are lovingly referred to in the gym. The traps are the muscles which connect the shoulder with the neck and with the shoulder blades.

Get Ready

Stand facing the mirror with your feet shoulder-length apart. Your knees should not be locked but should be bent slightly. With a dumbbell in each hand, your palms should be facing your thighs. Your back is straight and you should be looking yourself directly in the eyes of your image in the mirror.

The Exercise

Exhale and lift your shoulders toward your ears. As you look at yourself in the mirror your body language could read: "I don't know." Hold for one count. Inhale and ease the dumbbells toward the floor on a count of three-two-one. Feel the stretch as you finish the exhalation. Exhale and repeat.

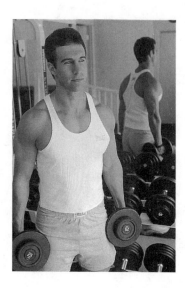 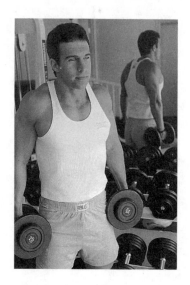

YOUR CHEST

Chest muscles are called pectoral muscles and are commonly referred to as "pecs." The muscle itself is comprised of long fibers shaped like strands of yarn. These strands of muscle hang like drapery from the base of the shoulder and connect along the entire breast bone. There are five basic areas of the chest that will be the focus of your attention and work. There is a top, middle, and bottom, an inside and outside area of the pectoral muscle. The upper portion lies just under each side of your collarbone. The bottom portion rises up on each side from the middle of the rib cage. The middle portion of the muscle takes up the majority of the surface area. The outer portion extends downward from the shoulder along the side of the chest and forms the bottom corner of the box. The inside portion of the muscle in a developed chest rises from the breast bone to form a valley of sorts.

It is essential to create well-rounded and equal development between all areas of the pectoral muscles. By virtue of what we do for a living, by partaking in certain activities, we naturally tend to have unbalanced development throughout the pectoral muscles. As we develop the chest, we begin to look better. The more evenly we develop this muscle, the more defined the musculature becomes, the better we look.

THE FLAT BENCH CHEST PRESS

This exercise is performed on a flat bench with dumbbells or with a bar. The flat bench chest press is designed to work the entire chest. It is best to begin by performing this exercise with dumbbells, to understand the importance of getting a deep starting point and to feel the fantastic stretch across the chest for each repetition. To facilitate this deep starting point, it is essential that the elbows be positioned to create the deepest possible stretch. The upper arm should be at a 90° angle with your torso at the beginning and end of each repetition. To eliminate the possibility of injuries, do not bounce during the stretch.

Get Ready

Sitting upright, bring one end of each dumbbell to the top of each knee. Push up with your legs and use the momentum to roll onto your back. Plant your feet firmly on the ground with your legs a comfortable distance apart. Bring the weights up so that your upper arms are at a 90° angle to your torso and the dumbbells are pointed in the same direction as your shoulders. Your upper arm is at a 90° angle with your forearm.

Breathe in and allow the elbows to point toward the ground as you lower your hands until they are almost even with your shoulders. **If you were doing this exercise with a bar, the bar would be across your collarbone.** Feel the stretch across your chest.

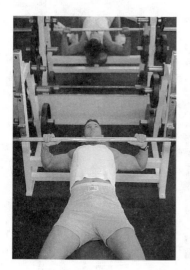

The Exercise

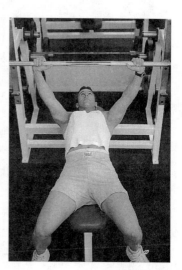

Exhale and drive the dumbbells straight up from the shoulders until the arms are fully extended but the elbows are not locked. Hold at the top of this movement for one count as you squeeze the chest muscles. Inhale and come down into your stretch on a count of six-five-four-three-two-one. Exhale and repeat the prescribed number of repetitions. Stretch after each set.

Stretch

If you happen to be working out with a partner, this stretch is a fantastic method to effectively stretch the chest muscles. Interlock your fingers and place your hands behind your head. Relax your shoulders and allow them drop as much as possible. With your partner behind you, have them pull your elbows back gently until you are getting a full stretch across the chest. Have them hold in this position or deepen the stretch for at least 30 seconds and no more than one minute.

If you are not working out with a partner, find a pole or bar that is immovable and at least 6 feet tall, stand in a doorway, or lean against the end of a wall. With your arm raised and at a 90° angle, place your right forearm along this immovable object. Turn your torso away from your raised arm until you feel this incredible stretch across one half of your chest. Hold this stretch for at least 30 seconds. Switch arms and perform this stretch on your left side for the exact same amount of time.

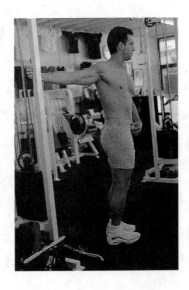

HOT POINT FITNESS

Although this exercise is similar to the flat bench press, the angle of attack is changed to target the upper region of the pectoral muscles. To get the fullest possible benefit from this exercise, it is vital to hold at the bottom of the movement and squeeze the chest muscles together at the top of the movement.

Get Ready

With a dumbbell in each hand, sit down on a bench that does not have a straight back, but is angled or reclined at a 45° angle. Plant your feet firmly on the ground with your legs a comfortable distance apart. Bring the weights up so that your upper arms are at a 90° angle to your torso and the dumbbells are pointed in the same direction as your shoulders. Your upper arm is at a 90° angle with your forearm.

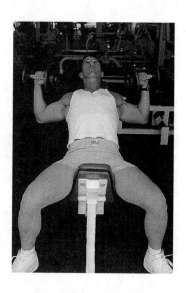

Breathe in and allow the elbows to reach backward as you lower your hands until they are almost even with the middle of your chest. If you were doing this exercise with a barbell, the bar would be just above your collarbone. Feel the stretch across your upper chest.

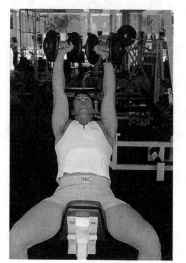

The Exercise

Exhale and drive the dumbbells straight up until the arms are fully extended but the elbows are not locked. The dumbells should be in a "V" shape. Hold at the top of this movement for one count as you squeeze the chest muscles. Inhale and come down into your stretch on a count of three-two-one and pause. Exhale and repeat the prescribed number of repetitions. Stretch after each set using the chest stretch.

DECLINED CHEST PRESS

This advanced exercise is designed to target the bottom of the pectoral muscles and has the secondary benefit of working the lower portion of the muscle group. Again, this is almost the exact same exercise as the flat bench chest press and the inclined chest press. The only difference is the angle of attack and the direction of the press.

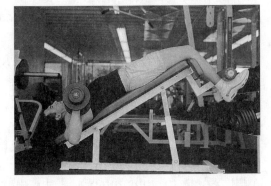

Get Ready

Some people experience a sense of light-headedness when they first attempt this exercise. Since we are not accustomed to hanging upside down, this position takes some getting used to. Try to work through the uneasiness and orient your body to this position. If the position is just too uncomfortable or makes you queasy, simply replace this exercise with the C Sweep.

With a dumbbell in each hand, hook your feet under the roll of the decline bench and gently lie down until your back has full contact with the bench.

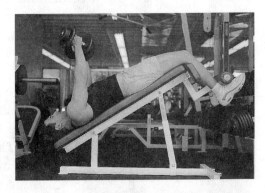

The Exercise

With your elbows at a 90° angle with your torso, bring the dumbbells down so that you feel a slight stretch across your chest. This stretch is essentially considered to be loading up for the press. Exhale and drive the weight straight up toward the ceiling until your arms are fully extended but the elbows are not locked. Turn your wrists slightly so the heels of your hands are pointing toward each other and the dumbbells are in the shape of a "V". Hold this position for one count, getting a full flex in the chest muscles. Inhale and come back into your stretch on a count of three-two-one and hold for one count. Repeat for the prescribed number of repetitions and stretch after each set using the chest stretch.

This exercise is designed to shape the pectoral muscles. This exercise is performed with dumbbells on either the flat bench, the incline bench, or the decline bench. You should choose a weight that is considerably lighter than the weight you used for the chest press. The object is again to achieve perfect or near-perfect technique. At the top of this exercise, I will ask you to squeeze your chest. On either side of your breast bone, the musculature will develop, creating sort of a valley that rises up to each side of the chest. If the muscles in your chest were large and highly developed, you would actually be attempting to squeeze these muscles together.

Get Ready

Plant your feet firmly on the ground with your legs a comfortable distance apart. Position your hands so that your knuckles are facing the ceiling and bring your elbows down so that they are below the bench and pointed toward the ground. Extend your hands to each side until your arms are to at least a 45°

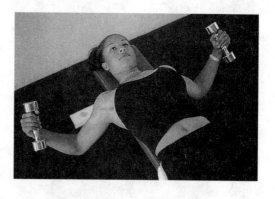

angle. You should be feeling a deep stretch across your chest. Your arms stay in this position as you. . .

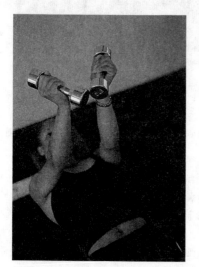

The Exercise

Exhale and drive the weight up, as if you were wrapping your arms over a barrel or a beach ball. When you are about halfway up, begin to straighten the elbows and let the dumbells come together as you reach the top of the movement. Bring the ends of the dumbbells together and form a "V" shape, and hold this position for one count as you squeeze the chest

INCLINE CHEST FLY

Start

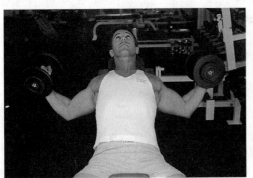

Finish

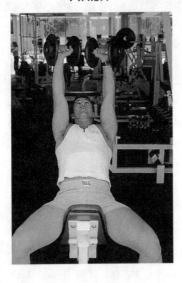

DECLINE CHEST FLY

Start

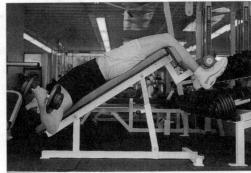

Finish

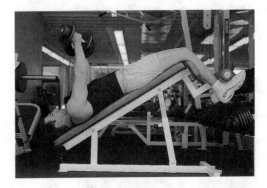

muscles together. Inhale and come down to your starting position on a count of three-two-one. Finish your exhalation for an additional two counts as you deepen the stretch across your chest. Really expose the chest, and DO NOT bounce when you are in this position. Exhale and repeat for the prescribed number of repetitions. Stretch after each set using the chest stretch.

PUSH UPS

The push up is an excellent chest exercise and is effective at working each section of the pectorals, if done properly. There are two basic ways to perform push-ups. In grade school we used to call them boy push-ups and girl push-ups, but in reality they are truly beginner push-ups and advanced push-ups.

BEGINNER PUSH-UPS

The Exercise

Lie face down on the floor. Cross your ankles, bend your knees, and lift your feet off the ground. Place your hands, palms down, underneath your shoulders. Exhale and push your body away from the floor so you are balancing on your hands and your knees. Do not let the buttocks go too high, but rather let your body form a straight line from your knees to your head. Inhale and come down on a count of three-two-one, until you almost touch the ground. Hold in this position for one count as you finish your inhalation. Exhale and repeat for the prescribed number of repetitions. Stretch after each set using the chest stretch.

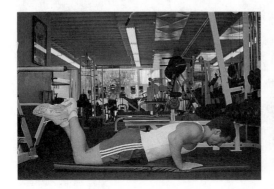 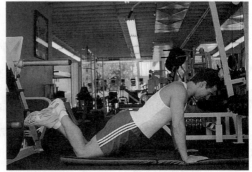

Create Muscle Strength at a Deeper Level . . . Quickly

ADVANCED PUSH-UPS

The Exercise

Lie face down on the floor. Curl your toes under your feet so you are resting on the balls of your feet. Simultaneously place your hands, palms down, under your shoulders. Exhale and push away from the floor, keeping your body in a straight

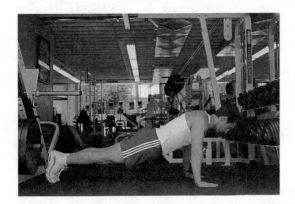

line from your head to your toes. Inhale and ease the body down on a count of three-two-one until your chest almost touches the floor. Hold this position for one count. Exhale and repeat for the prescribed number of repetitions. Stretch after each set using the chest stretch.[3]

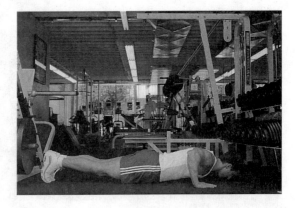

[3]After you are able to complete three sets of the advanced push-up, you may experiment with your hand position. If you are performing three sets, begin with the advanced push-up described above. For the next set place your hands, palms down, just below your neck and make a triangle out of your thumbs and index fingers. For the next set place your hands, palms down, just outside your shoulders. Changing your hand position for each set will ensure that different parts of the chest are being targeted.

HOT POINT FITNESS

This exercise is named after the machine you will use to perform it. Although this exercise will work the entirety of the chest muscles, the pec deck is designed to work the entirety of the chest, and specifically target the innermost portion of the pectoral muscles, which run up and down the length of your breast bone. The only drawback to this machine is that it is not geared for all body types. I have noticed that shorter people will not fit properly when seated in most of these machines. If you happen to fall into this category, simply take the pad you perform sit-ups on and place it against the back seat cushion.

Get Ready

Sit in the chair provided by the machine. Press your feet against the footrest to move the bars forward. Place your forearms on the pads provided so that your forearms are at a 90° angle in relation to your biceps. *Allow*

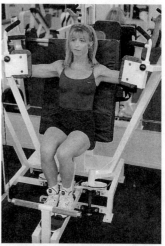

your wrists to bend backward so that only your forearm is touching the pad.

The Exercise

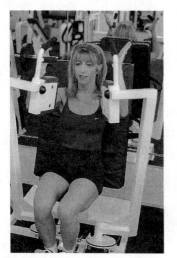

Exhale and bring your arms together, leading with your elbows, NOT your hands. As your arms come together, really squeeze, and hold this position for two counts to get a full flex in your chest muscles as you finish your

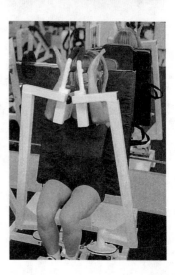

exhalation. Inhale, and on a count of three-two-one, let the arms come back to the starting position. You will feel a nice stretch across your chest. Exhale and repeat the prescribed number of repetitions. Stretch after each set.

Stretch

After completing each set, press the footrest to hold the bar out as far as it will go, and keep the bar in this position. Release your arms and shake the blood back into circulation. Put your arms back on the forearm pad and slowly release the footrest on the machine, allowing for a deep and full stretch across your chest. Maintain this continuous stretch for at least 30 seconds.

The "C" sweep is designed to target and work the outer border of the pectoral muscles. This exercise is performed with dumbbells on the flat bench. The basic movement for this exercise is to trace a "C" around your torso with each hand. Achieving a total chest workout with this exercise requires perfect or near perfect technique.

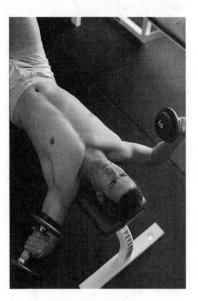

The key is to maximize the movement at the starting and ending points of the C sweep. The exercise begins with a deep stretch, to hit the top of the pecs with pinpoint accuracy, and ends by flexing the chest muscles to develop the bottom portion of the chest muscles.

Get Ready

Lie down on a flat bench with a dumbbell in each hand. Bend your legs and place the soles of your feet on the bench, so that your knees are pointing toward the ceiling. With your elbows pointed toward the ground, bring your hands slightly higher than the shoulders so the dumbbells are even with your ears and your knuck-

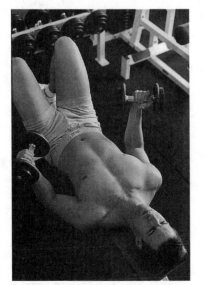

les are facing the ceiling. You will now trace a C-shape with each hand.

The Exercise

Exhale and, without letting the hands rise any higher, use the chest muscles to sweep the dumbbells to the level of your waist in the pattern of an arc. Continuing the exhalation and the arc movement, gradually turn the wrists as your arms pass the waist and continue to trace the bottom of the "C." During the last portion of this movement, where you are finishing the "C", allow your hands to rise slightly. With the palms facing in the direction of your head, hold this position as you feel the bottom of the pectoral muscles flex. Inhale and reverse the "C" on a count of four-three-two-one. Feel the deep stretch across your chest as you finish your inhalation. Exhale and repeat the prescribed number of repetitions. Stretch after each set using the chest stretch.

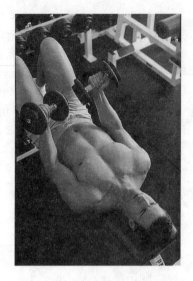

YOUR SHOULDERS

The shoulders are divided into three sections— front, middle, and rear. Anatomically, this muscle group is called the deltoid. In gym lingo, it is commonly referred to as your "delts." The deltoids are muscles that look like a scallop shell or, when under extreme strain, look like the fingers on a hand. Men and women will work this muscle group a little differently. Men usually will prefer to create mass, giving the shoulders a wider look. Women typically look to create more definition in this area, which accentuates and flatters the upper arm.

For men and women, the rear portion of the shoulder is greatly underdeveloped. Unless you row a boat several times per week, there is probably nothing that you do in your everyday life that works this area. You can prevent some fairly painful physical problems if you develop the musculature in this area. I'll give you an example. Stand straight up. Lift your arms straight out to the sides like you were stopping traffic in both directions. Now let your arms drop. Ideally your hands will come to rest just inside the hip bones, with their palms facing each other. Most men will come to a resting position with their hands facing forward and their palms facing to the rear. What this indicates is a muscular imbalance. The muscles in the front have become overdeveloped and the muscles in the rear are underdeveloped. As a consequence, the shoulders have effectively rolled over. The more the shoulders roll to the front, the greater the problems with posture. The more unbalanced your posture, the greater the risk for injury and ailments. Typically, posture-related ailments take the form of back problems, shoulder aches, and eventually lead to a stooped or hunched-over appearance as you advance in age. As the imbalance becomes more pronounced and extreme, it can even cause serious circulation issues. These can often be relieved, or in some instances eliminated, by correcting posture. The deltoid muscles are the key to correcting this posture problem. For athletically inclined people, even on the professional level, this imbalance can prevent you from attaining your best game. For aesthetic and overall health reasons, it is imperative to attain muscular balance in this area.

W SHOULDERS

The W shoulders is tailored to work all three areas of the deltoid muscle. This exercise is performed with a pair of dumbbells and is the most effective exercise for working the muscle to 100% of its ability. If you have worked out before or even do so regularly, you will want to use a fairly light weight for this exercise. If you can lift 50-pound dumbbells over your head, you will want to use 15-pound weights for this particular exercise—it is that drastic. Believe me, this Hot Point exercise will make you feel like your shoulders are on fire.

Get Ready

With a dumbbell in each hand, sit facing the mirror on a bench with a straight back to support your spine. With your legs spread a comfortable distance apart, plant your feet firmly on the ground. With your palms facing toward your shoulders, lower the dumbbells to shoulder level, as if the weight were an extension of the shoulder. Your elbows should be pointed straight toward the ground, and when you look in the mirror, you are in the shape of a "W."

The Exercise

Exhale and drive your hands straight up toward the ceiling until the shape of your arms look like a "U" or a goal post. Hold this point for one count. Release back into the shape of a "W" on a count of three-two-one and hold for one count. Exhale and repeat for the prescribed number of repetitions. Stretch after each set.

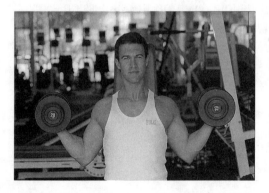 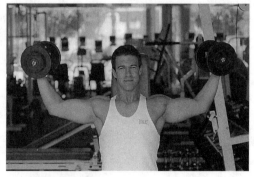

Stretch

Stand up and face the mirror. Extend your right arm straight out in front of you, and bring it across your chest. Place your left hand on the elbow of your right arm. Relax the right shoulder, and let it drop down. Use the left hand to gently hug the right arm to your chest. As you breathe in and out, allow this stretch to deepen. Maintain this stretch for at least 30 seconds before repeating on the left side.

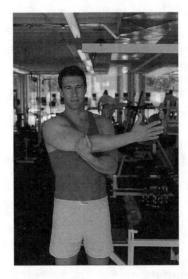

GOAL POST

This exercise is designed to work all three areas of the deltoid muscle, as the shoulder joint rotates. The only joint that moves in this exercise is the shoulder joint. The rest of the body remains fixed and rigid.

Get Ready

Sit in a straight-backed bench facing the mirror. With a dumbbell in each hand, bring your arms into a 90° angle with the dumbbells toward the ceiling so that when you look in the mirror, your arms are in the position of a football goal post. Use only the shoulder joint to move.

The Exercise

Inhale and allow the dumbbells to slowly drop toward the floor on a count of three-two-one, until your forearms are parallel with the floor. Hold for one count as you finish your inhalation. Exhale and bring the dumbbells to an upright position on a count of one-two-three, until you are in the shape of a goal post. Inhale and repeat for the prescribed number of repetitions. Stretch after each set using the deltoid stretch.

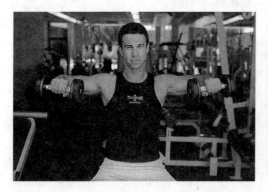 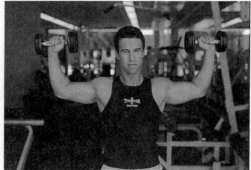

The movement for this exercise is very similar to that of a bird in flight. This is the most basic exercise for the rear portion of the deltoid. The delt wing is performed using two dumbbells. Again, low weight and proper technique are the keys.

Get Ready

With a dumbbell in each hand, place your chest against the backrest of the incline bench. Either kneel on the seat or place your feet firmly on the ground. Scoot up so that your chin is over the top of the chair.

The Exercise

With your knees pointed toward the floor, exhale and bring the weights straight out to the side until they are almost parallel to your shoulders. Hold for one count. Inhale on a count of three-two-one and bring the weights back down until they are back in the starting position. Inhale and complete the prescribed number of repetitions. Stretch after each set using the deltoid stretch.

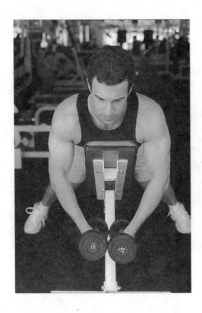

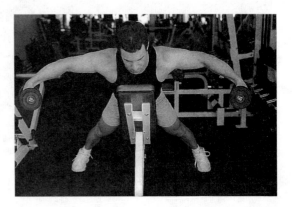

Create Muscle Strength at a Deeper Level . . . Quickly

LATERAL RAISE

This exercise is designed to work the middle portion of the deltoid muscle. Again, this exercise is performed with two dumbbells. The key to this exercise is proper hand placement.

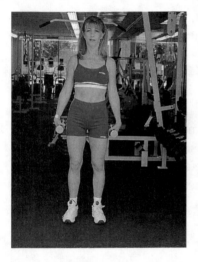

Get Ready

With a dumbbell in each hand, stand and face the mirror. Your legs should be spread shoulder-width apart, with your feet flat on the ground and firmly planted, and kness bent slightly. Turn your wrists in like you were carrying a suitcase.

The Exercise

Exhale and bring the weight up, so that the top of your wrists are facing the ceiling and your arms are in a straight line with your shoulders. Hold this position for one count as you finish your exhalation. Inhale and slowly release the arms back down to the starting position on a count of three-two-one. Regroup as you exhale and inhale. Exhale and repeat the prescribed number of repetitions. Stretch after each set using the deltoid stretch.

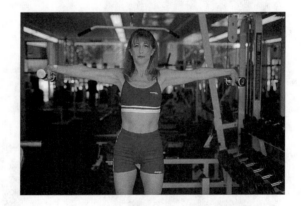

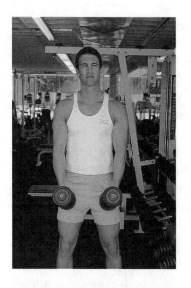

This exercise is designed to work the front portion of your deltoid muscles. The front raise is performed using two dumbbells, and the movement of this exercises is very much like tracing a box with your dumbbells.

Get Ready

With a dumbbell in each hand, stand facing the mirror. Your hands should be in the same position as they would be if you were carrying two suitcases. Spread your legs a comfortable distance apart and plant your feet firmly on the ground bending your knees slightly.

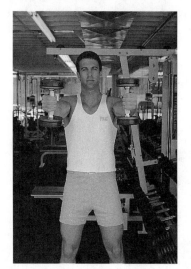

The Exercise

Exhale and, with your arms extended, lift the weights straight up in front of you until your arms are coming straight out from your shoulders and your fists are aimed at the mirror. Turn your wrists so your palms are facing the floor and bring the dumbbells together until they almost touch. Hold for one count. Inhale, turn your wrists back to their original position, and bring the arms down on a count of three-two-one, until the weights are just above your knees with your arms extended. Exhale and repeat for the prescribed number of repetitions. Stretch after each set using the deltoid stretch.

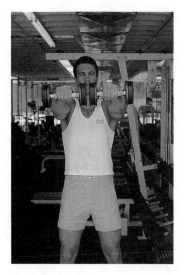

YOUR TRICEPS

There are three connection points where the muscle attaches to the skeletal system. If you extend your arm and flex your triceps, well-developed musculature will be in almost the shape of a horseshoe. To maximize any tricep exercise, it is vital to isolate the muscle being used as much as possible. With all of the exercises focusing on the triceps, the only joint that will move will be your elbow. Not only is it vital to keeping all other body parts in a fixed position, but the elbows themselves must remain fixed as well, and not be allowed to move in and out.

Men and women concentrate on the triceps for slightly different reasons. Men should concentrate on this area at least as much as they would the biceps, as developing this muscle makes the arm balanced and creates a much fuller-looking arm. If size and mass is your goal, pay particular attention to developing the triceps. For women, this is the exact area to concentrate on. You will be working this area with many repetitions and a relatively light weight, so there is no need to worry about overdeveloping these muscles. The object is to create definition. It is precisely the definition that you create in these muscles which create a sculpted and toned arm. Defining these muscles will make your arms look thinner, and working these muscles will also eliminate any perceivable jiggle when you wave.

The tricep extension is designed to work the inside and outside portion of the tricep muscle. The only portion of your body that is actually moving is your elbow joint. Think of this joint as if it were a hinge on a door. The door does not wobble, the wall does not weave back and forth, only the hinge moves.

Get Ready

This tricep exercise utilizes two dumbbells. As with any excercise using dumbbells, always work to the weaker arm. This means only do as many repititions with the dominant arm as you can perform with the weaker arm. The point is to catch the weaker arm up to the dominant arm, and then develop both arms together. After both arms are at this level and have been so for some time, you can rotate to perform this excercise using a bar.

With a dumbbell in each hand, lie down on a flat bench with your eyes looking at the ceiling. Your feet should be a comfortable length apart and planted firmly and flat against the ground.

The Excercise

Bring the dumbbells just above the very top of your forehead, and turn your wrists slightly so that the heads of the dumbbells nearest your head almost touch. Your elbows should be pointing toward the ceiling. Your thumb should be nearest to

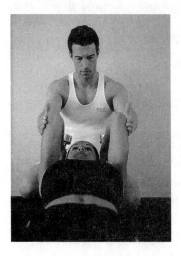 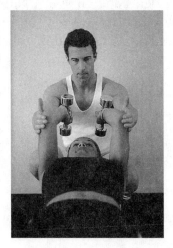 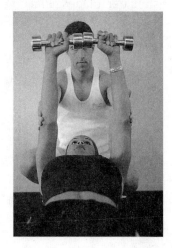

your head, and the heel of your hand should be pointing away from your face. (If you are performing this excercise with the bar, your palms should be facing away from your face.) Bring your elbows close together, so they are shoulder-width apart. Exhale and drive the weight up until you are pointing the weights at the place where the wall meets the ceiling. Do not fully extend the arms, as it would

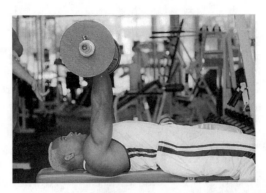

take all the pressure off the triceps. Rotate your wrists until your palms are facing away from you, and hold for one count. Inhale on a count of three-two-one as you slowly bring the weights to the top of your forehead. This negative movement should remain very controlled. Come back too quickly and you will learn how this excercise got the nickname "braincrusher." Stretch after each set.

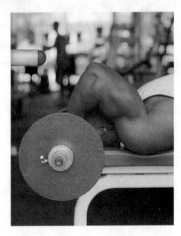

Stretch

Stand or sit at the end of the bench and place your right elbow between your shoulder blades. Place your left hand on your right elbow and come as close as

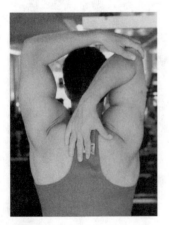

you can to pointing your elbow straight up toward the ceiling. Continue this stretch for all excercises involving the triceps.

The overhead tricep extension can be an awkward exercise for some. It is important not to be overly macho in choosing your weight. Start light on this exercise and work your way up over time. The overhead tricep extension is performed with a dumbbell and is designed to totally isolate the tricep muscle. It will work them harder that they have ever been worked.

Get Ready

Sit on a flat bench with your feet firmly planted on the floor. With a dumbbell in your left hand, bring the weight directly behind your head, and position the dumbbell so that it is parallel with your spine. Your left elbow should be pointed toward the ceiling, and your right bicep should be in a direct line with your right shoulder. You may place your right hand on your left elbow to prevent that elbow from moving side to side. The only joint that will move is your elbow. The shoulders, torso, and upper arms remain in a fixed position 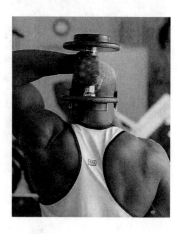 throughout the exercise. The point is to isolate the triceps as much as possible.

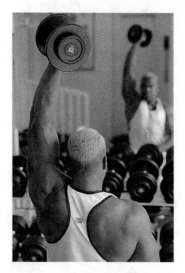

The Exercise

Exhale and drive the weight up. Inhale and release the elbow joint back to the starting position on a count of three-two-one. Inhale and regroup as you feel the stretch. Exhale and repeat for the specified number of repetitions. Switch to the right side, complete the specified number of repetitions, and you will have completed one set. Stretch the triceps after each set using the tricep stretch.

BENCH DIPS

This exercise uses the weight of your body rather that weights to target all three areas of your triceps.

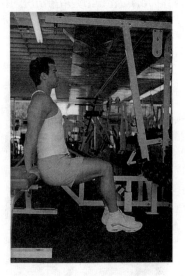

Get Ready

Sit on a flat bench with both of your legs on one side. Bring your hands close to your buttocks and grip the edge of the bench, so that your elbows are pointing away from you. Walk your feet out slightly and plant them firmly on the ground. Slide off the bench until your legs are in a 90° angle and you are supporting your weight with your arms. Keep your back straight, your shoulders pressed down, and make certain to not let your elbows point out to the sides throughout this exercise.

The Exercise

Inhale and lower your butt toward the floor on a count of three-two-one until your elbows will not allow you to go any lower. Exhale and drive your body up, pressing your elbows toward each other to maintain their proper position. Straighten your arms until your elbows almost lock. Inhale and repeat the prescribed number of repetitions. Stretch after each set using the tricep stretch.

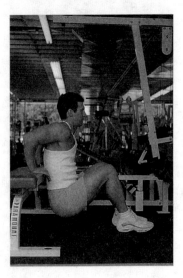

The tricep push-down is performed on the machine utilizing the overhead cable. There are a number of different bars to choose from and attach to this cable. If you use a straight bar today, use a bent bar the next time you perform this exercise. Always make a note of the bar last used and choose a different bar the next time you perform it. The most important aspects of this exercise are elbow placement and

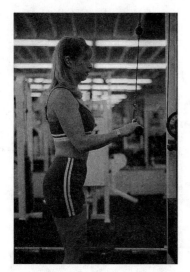

proper wrist movement. Following the directions for these body parts will allow you to keep pressure on the triceps and to achieve the maximum results from this exercise.

Get Ready

Stand straight up facing the machine, with your knees slightly bent. Place your hands, palms down, on the bar in front of you. Bring the bar down slightly so that your wrists are straight and your elbows are just in front of your stomach. Pretend that there is a brace that keeps your elbows this exact distance apart, and do not let them stray from this position throughout the exercise.

The Exercise

Exhale and drive the weight down, turning your wrists as you go, until your arms are fully extended but not locked. Hold this position for one count. Your knuckles should be pointed straight toward the ceiling, your wrist in a similar position to dribbling a basketball. Inhale and bring the weight back up to the starting position on a count of three-two-one, straightening your wrists as the bar comes up. Exhale and repeat until you complete the prescribed number of repetitions. Stretch after each set using the tricep stretch.

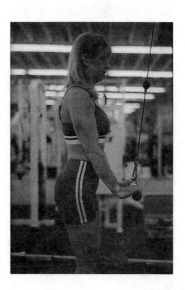

Create Muscle Strength at a Deeper Level . . . Quickly

TRICEP KICKBACK WITH A TWIST

This exercise is designed to work both the inside and the outside of the tricep muscle, and is created to confuse the muscle with each repetition. It demands that the triceps be isolated, meaning that you will not swing your body to move the weight. Your elbow and wrist will be the only joints which actually move. Because this exercise is a stellar example of momentumless training, as it isolates the triceps and works the entirety of the muscle, it is perhaps the finest all-around exercise you could perform for this muscle group.

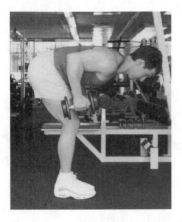

Get Ready

With a dumbbell in each hand, stand facing the mirror. With your back straight and knees bent, lean toward the mirror until your torso is parallel with the ground. Raise your elbows until they are parallel with your torso, so that your arms are at a 90° angle and your knuckles are facing the floor. You are now in the position of a skier headed downhill. The basic movement in this exercise would be like propelling yourself down hill by using your ski poles. Press your upper arms tightly against the rib cage and do not let them move for the du-

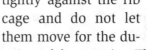

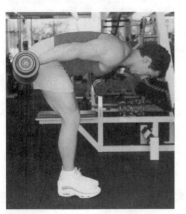

ration of the exercise. This will further serve the isolation of the tricep muscles.

The Exercise

From this "skiing" position, use the elbow as a hinge. Exhale and drive the weights behind you until your arms are fully extended. Hold in this position for one count as you rotate your wrists so that your thumbs are facing each other and your palms are facing the ceiling. Finish your exhalation and rotate the wrists back to the neutral position. Inhale and slowly release your hands back to the starting position on a count of three-two-one. Exhale to drive the weights back. Hold for one count. Turn the wrists so that your thumbs are pointing away from your body and your palms are facing the floor. Inhale to come back down to your starting point on a count of three-two-one. With each repetition, alternate between turning the wrists in and out. Repeat for the prescribed number of sets. Stretch after each set using the tricep stretch.

YOUR BICEPS

This particular muscle connects to the skeletal system at two points. Your goal is to create an elongated bicep, and to accomplish this will demand strict technique. There are usually two strategies for developing this muscle. Which one you choose is usually determined by your sex. If you are looking to create mass, or increasing the size of the bicep, you will truly want to work this muscle to exhaustion with heavy weight and fewer repititions. To achieve greater definition will require that you simply work with a greater number of repetitions and less weight.

The curl is the basic bicep exercise. This exercise will be performed with two dumbbells and the weight of your choice. Strict technique is vital to maximizing this exercise. There are two important factors to the movement. The first is correct elbow placement. While you can perform this exercise from a standing or seated position, it is vital that the bicep muscle be isolated so that you can ensure that only this muscle is involved in the movement.[4]

Get Ready

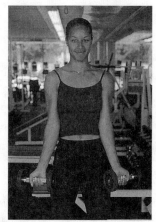

To facilitate this isolation, your elbow should be at your side, tucked into the smaller bottom-most ribs. Make certain that the elbow does not move from this fixed position. DO NOT swing the body to get the weight up. Use only the bicep muscle. BRING IT—DON'T SWING IT! The second important factor concerns the elongation of the bicep muscle. When most people perform this exercise, they do not get full development of the entire muscle. You must make certain that you bring the weight all the way down so

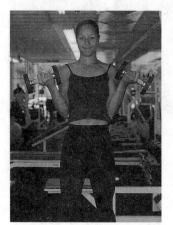

that you can fully stretch this muscle out. Failing to bring the weight down fully in this manner means that you are only working a small portion of the bicep, or about 35% of the entire muscle, making for an uneven, bulky, and malformed muscle. If you have proper technique, you can create an aesthetic of a well-defined and elongated arm.

With a dumbbell in each hand, stand facing the mirror with your palms facing forward. Your elbow should be just above your hip bone and will remain fixed throughout the exercise.

The Exercise

Exhale and bring the dumbbell up about 3/4 of the way toward your shoulder, turning your wrists so that the heel of your hand is pointing toward your chin.

Hold this position for one count as you finish your exhalation and get the fullest possible contraction in the biceps. Inhale and release the weight all the way down on a count of three-two-one. Feel the stretch at the bottom of the exercise. Exhale and repeat.

Stretch

Stand facing the mirror. Extend your arms straight out from your shoulders with your fingers pointing toward the ceiling, as if you were standing in the middle of the street stopping traffic in both directions. With your arms and hands locked in this position, rotate the arms so that your fingers are now pointing away from the mirror (or even toward the floor). Lock your arms in this position and rotate the wrist so that your hands are now in the traffic-stopping position. Feel this stretch the biceps and the forearm.

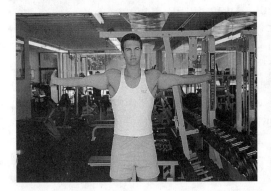 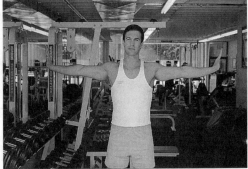

---

[4]As you become more advanced, and you are able to use the same weight and complete the same number of repetitions with each arm, you may use a bar or the cable machine instead of the dumbbells.

This exercise is performed with a dumbbell and is an ideal exercise for completely isolating the bicep muscle. The point of the exercise is to get a full contraction from the entire bicep muscle. Like "the curl," you do not want to swing the weight or use your back muscle to move the weight. Isolation is the key to success.

Get Ready

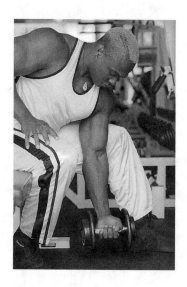

Sit on a flat bench facing the mirror. Your feet should be slightly wider than shoulder-width apart, and the dumbbell should be on the floor between your feet. Bend at the waist and place your right elbow inside your right knee. Place your left arm on top of your left knee, creating a 90° angle with your left arm. Lower your right arm down toward the floor until it is fully extended, and grip the dumbbell.

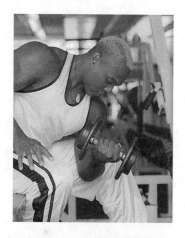

The Exercise

Keeping the left elbow in a fixed position against the knee, exhale and bring the weight up 3/4 of the way toward your left shoulder. When the weight reaches this point, twist your wrist so that your thumb is turning toward the mirror and the heel of your hand is turning toward your body. Finish your exhalation and hold this position for one count. Feel the entire bicep muscle in full contraction. Release the wrist and lower the weight on a count of three-two-one until your arm is fully extended. Feel the stretch throughout the bicep. Perform the designated number of repetitions and repeat on the right side. Stretch after each set for at least 30 seconds using the bicep stretch.

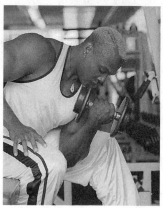

HAMMER CURLS

The hammer curl is performed with a dumbbell in each hand. This exercise is designed to work the outside portion of the bicep and will have secondary benefits for the upper portion of your forearm.

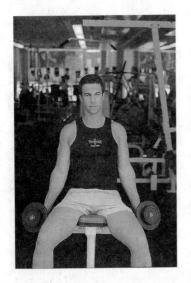

Get Ready

Sit on a bench or stand facing the mirror, arms at your sides, with a dumbbell in each hand so that your knuckles are facing the floor. Press your elbows into your torso, and keep them fixed throughout the exercise. This elbow placement will ensure the necessary isolation for the muscles you are working

The Exercise

Keeping the wrist and upper arm in a fixed position, exhale and bring both dumbbells 3/4 of the way toward the shoulders. The knuckle of the index finger and thumb are now facing your shoulder, and you are in the position of a ready boxer. Hold for one count as you reach the top. Moving only with your elbow joint, exhale and release the dumbbells back down to the starting position on a count of three-two-one. Fully extend the arm to feel the stretch through your bicep and repeat for the specified number of repetitions. Stretch after completing each set for at least 30 seconds.

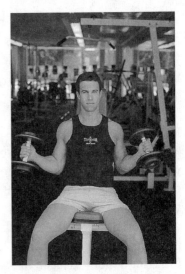

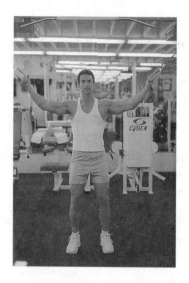

This exercise is performed on the cable machine. I personally find it to be one of the most intense exercises for the biceps, and you just may find that this will exhaust your muscles like no other. To facilitate this exercise you should place the hand grip attachments on the upper connection point on both sides of the machine.

Get Ready

After taking hold of each grip, take a few steps out in front of the machine so that there is significant tension in the cable. With your arms outstretched, your hands should now be behind you. Stand tall with your spine straight and your head upright.

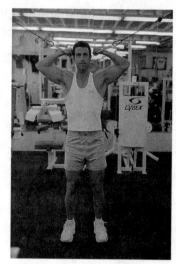

The Exercise

Exhale and bring your fists to a point just behind your ears. Hold this position for one count as the biceps flex. Inhale and allow the hands to go back into your starting position on a count of three-two-one. Exhale and repeat the prescribed number of repetitions, stretching with the bicep stretch after every set.[5]

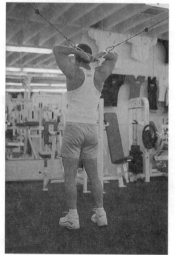

---

[5]As you become more advanced, bring your knuckles together behind your head, without tilting your head forward.

YOUR FOREARMS

The muscles of the forearm are long strands which reach from your wrists to your elbows. These are very important muscles for gripping objects and are often a point of focus for the elderly and athletes such as wrestlers, and baseball and hockey players, where the grip on another person, the bat, or stick is an integral part of the game. If this area is in need of rehabilitation or if the forearms are of particular concern to you, simply insert this exercise at the end of every other workout day.

If you are looking to improve your grip, perhaps one set will be plenty for this muscle group. If you are looking to create definition, one or two sets will be sufficient. If you are looking to create mass and get forearms like Popeye, perform at least 4 sets of this exercise.

FOREARM CABLE CURLS

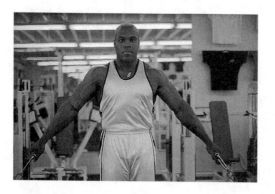

This exercise is performed on the cable machine and is designed to work your entire forearm muscle. Place the hand grips at the lowest connection point on each side of the cable machine.

Get Ready

With a grip in each hand, stand in the center of the cable machine. The only portion of your body that is moving throughout this exercise is your wrist. Extend your arms with your palms facing the floor. Your arms will remain in this fixed position for the remainder of the exercise.

The Exercise

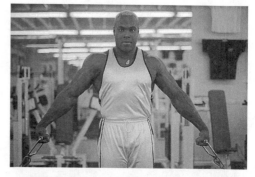

Curl your wrists in toward your body so that your knuckles are pointing toward the floor. Hold this position for two counts. Repeat this movement and perform 20 repetitions. With your hands and arms in the same position, curl your wrists out away from your body so that your knuckles are pointing toward the ceiling. Repeat this movement and perform 20 repetitions.

Stretch

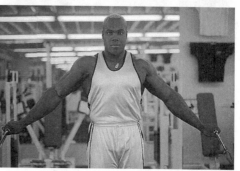

With your right arm in the curl position and your palm open and facing you, place the fingers of your left hand across the fingers on your right hand. Extend your right elbow and use the left hand to bend the right fingers toward your body. Feel this stretch from your wrist to your shoulder. Hold for at least 30 seconds and repeat on the other side.

5

Fuel Your Body for Optimum Performance

Hot Point Nutrition and Eating to Win

The point is to have the old you melt into the new you that you are working so diligently to create. Your diet is the foundation of the pyramid. The consistency of your diet will determine how rapidly you see results. The point of Hot Point Nutrition is to speed the metabolism and make it burn calories at a white-hot pace. To facilitate this process, you must be acutely vigilant about what you are putting in your body, and also by what you are fueling all of this added activity with.

Dieting has become an American obsession. Diet and nutrition are *the* most talked about topics in our popular culture. You cannot walk through a grocery store, turn on the TV, listen to the radio, or open your e-mail without being bombarded with the latest fad diet that promises a thinner you. Most of these diets are not worth the paper that they are printed on. When discussing the issues of weight loss and weight gain, I feel that it is important to break the cycle that most people seem to be stuck in. It is my opinion that the negative connotation that most of us feel about our weight has to do with the way in which we measure it.

Weight is a problem for many of us. Some of us really have to watch every bite that we eat, and with much suffering and sacrifice, are able to lose a little when we look at our weight on the scale. Some of us tried every diet known to man, and still nothing works. There are also people on the other extreme. These people have to try very hard to maintain their weight. A little slip, too much work, too many family events, too much running around, and they are dropping weight like nobody's business. For them, gaining weight would be a dream come true. Because most of us are somewhere between these two extremes (wanting to add a little here and take off a little there), it is important that we understand both ends of the spectrum to really figure out what will work best for you.

Because weight loss and weight gain are emotionally charged issues for some, it is a wise strategy to draw your attention away from the scale. The scale is the most frequently used instrument of our ability to measure our progress, and it is precisely that progress which needs to be redefined. To redefine weight and eliminate all the emotional baggage that comes with the scale, we should examine what the scale tells us.

Let's be realistic. . . . Do you really care how much you weigh on the scale, or are you more interested in dropping a few dress sizes, fitting into your "skinny" pants, or being the same size you were way back when? If you were 5 pounds heavier than you are today but were three sizes smaller, would you complain? Let's put it to you another way. With Hot Point Fitness, you are going to be lifting weights and doing aerobic exercise. By performing exactly these kinds of exercises, you are going to be increasing the density (but not necessarily the size) of the muscle. Muscle weighs about two times more than fat, so it is entirely possible that your weight may actually go up but your size will go down.

Weight Is Not the Point

The scale is a misleading and inaccurate indicator of what is going on with your body. Weight has little to do with your situation. When you step on the scale, you are seeing three separate and wholly different aspects of the total picture. When you step on the scale, you are weighing muscle, fat, and other important body parts, such as water, hair, organs, and bone. If you could actually separate these three distinct categories, you would see a much clearer picture of what was actually happening in your body and how to change it. If these divergent bodily properties could be separated into categories, this would be very useful information.

Instead of guessing, you could determine how much muscle or bone density you have gained and how much fat you have lost. Such a measurement is not a mere flight of fancy, but is available and accessible to everyone.

Body-Fat Percentage

The body-fat percentage measurement is absolutely essential, and will give you accurate information to better assess where you are at this very moment in the transformational process, and also to mark your progress as you continue your journey. There are many methods to perform this measurement, and they range in price from $5 to $15,000. The most accurate, accessible, and cost-efficient way to have your body fat measured is by a trained professional using a device called a skin-fold caliper. The professional will typically take measurements on three to five different parts of your body and use the caliper to measure how much fat is underneath the skin. After taking your total weight on the scale, they then equate these measurements with a mathematical formula to determine your body-fat percentage. Often you can have this measurement taken at the gym, by a licensed nutritionist, accredited personal trainers, or by many doctors. This test should cost anywhere from $15-$35 to have performed, and the results will be an invaluable tool for you. If you should have any difficulty in finding a facility that measures body fat, you can call the American Council on Exercise at (800) 825–3636 for a personal trainer in your area. IDEA FIT also can refer you to a trainer in your area that can take this measurement, and they can be reached at (800) 999-4332, or you may use their web site locator at www.ideafit.com. When this measurement is taken, you will see what your total weight is, how much of that total weight is composed of fat, and how much is muscle. Instead of stepping on the scale every day to check your progress, have your body-fat percentage measured every few weeks. Learning the ratios of fat and lean muscle mass is vital information, which can truly change your perspective and approach when you address this emotional topic. This vital information is the basis for creating the ideal nutritional plan for you. The entire Hot Point Diet is based upon this information, and it is important that you have this measurement taken before you begin your nutritional program. Promise yourself that you will have this measurement taken before you finish this chapter. It is vital to determining how much food you should be eating. Creating the ideal nutritional plan for you will mean giving the muscles and bones all the nutrients they need and denying the portion of your body that is made up of fat.

Remember, no matter what your goal, the objective is to get and keep your body-fat percentage as low as possible. To do this, it is again important that you create a strategy to outthink your body. The body does not like to part with fat. Humans have survived as long as we have because the body is equipped with tremendously effective survival mechanisms. Fat is the *ultimate* survival tool. The most basic survival mode is to prevent starvation.

We must trick the body into never shifting into a survival mode. When we eat, the body utilizes our food very efficiently. Like an energy-efficient machine, our bodies use the minimum amount of nutrients to fuel our activity and place the rest in a reserve tank, our body fat. Our fat then becomes a vast reservoir of reserve fuel. However, this reserve is regarded by the body as an emergency source. Our bodies are wired to equate fat loss with death. When you go without eating, your body thinks it is starving. So in addition to NOT expending any of the fat reserve, you will lose muscle tissue and bone density. These are all desirous entities, which promote your physical and mental health, have the ability to actually burn body fat, and offset the percentage of body fat. So, it is most advantageous to keep bone and muscle density. To avoid this phenomenon, you never, ever, want to let your body think it is starving.

We often fail ourselves when we either eat too much or too little. When we eat too much, the body only uses what it needs and then saves the rest for later. When we eat too little, the body shifts into a starvation mode and will not expend fat. When we finally do eat, the body stores most of the food into our fat because it is unsure when and if it will ever be fed again. This is exactly why most diets fail. If you are on a low-calorie diet or a diet that is made up of a particular food group, the body thinks that it is starving. Before tapping into the fuel reserve, the body eats up muscle and organ tissue. This means that the percentage of your total body weight made up of fat is actually *increasing*. That's right, you are actually getting **fatter**! When you do eat, the body takes the food and hoards it in the fat cells, so you get **fatter still**. The weight loss you are seeing on the scale may actually be a loss in muscle, bone, and water, and very little (if any) of that loss on the scale will be from a loss of fat. This starvation mode becomes a vicious cycle, and after you quit the diet out of disappointment, your body is still in a survival mode. To avoid this phenomenon and effectively break the cycle, you must feed yourself regularly so that your body can trust that it will be taken care of. Remember, you want to provide the body with enough fuel to drive your activity, but not enough to store in a reserve tank.

Figuring Out How Much You Need

To emotionally detach yourself even further from the weight issue, think of it this way: creating the proper nutritional program basically boils down to a math problem. By all means, emotionally detach from this subject even further by making the weight issue solely and entirely about some numbers on a page. How emotional can math be? You have already measured your body-fat percentage, and now you know how much of your total weight is made up of the things you want more of (muscle and bone) and the thing you want less of (fat). Because you are starting a consistent program using aerobic and weight training, you will be creating more lean muscle mass, and because this muscle will weigh more, you will consequently have a lower percentage of your total body weight that is made up of fat. By implementing a sound nutritional program, you can tip these scales even further by actually decreasing the amount of fat you are carrying around with you.

Remember, what you want to do is provide the muscle and bone with enough food to fuel it throughout the day and limit the amount of nutrients you are providing to the fat. Before creating your nutritional plan, ask yourself these questions: 1) Do you want to increase size? You may feel that you are lean enough, but what you are really striving for is putting on muscle mass. 2) Do you want to maintain your same weight but create muscular definition? You may feel that weight is not your primary concern, but you do want to lose some inches around the middle and create tone and strength in the musculature. 3) Do you want to lose fat? You may want to shed a considerable amount of fat and tone and shape the musculature that resides underneath.

It is now time to put this information into perspective and create a nutritional program that is ideal for your goals. The first determination that needs to be made in your particular math problem centers upon your body-fat percentage. By now you should have had this measurement taken. Mark down this information in the space provided.

Total Weight	_____
Body-fat percentage	_____
Pounds of fat	_____
Pounds of muscle, bone, hair, organs, and water	_____

Remember that this is just math, and it's a simple equation. If you want to remove fat from your body, you will want to burn more calories than you take in.

One pound of fat contains 3,500 calories. Calories are simply a unit of measurement representing the amount of stuff our bodies use as fuel. When you are exercising at an aerobic level for at least 25 minutes, you will burn calories to fuel that activity. Approximately half of those calories will be drawn from the food you have eaten, and the other half will be drawn from your reserve tank, or body fat. If you eat 2,000 calories per day, and do so many minutes of aerobic exercise, that burns X amount of calories. That means that half of those calories are being extracted from your fat to be used as fuel. You *do* need to eat to fuel the body and the mind, so let's figure out what and how much you should be eating to achieve your goals.

Determining how much you need to eat, and creating a way of eating that you can adhere to for the rest of your life, is all about balance. Just as you want the right thigh to be the same size as the left thigh, just as you want the calves and biceps to be the same size, you want to create a sense of proportion in your meals. By creating meals that have the proper balance of protein, carbohydrate, and fat, you will hasten your physical transformation. By practicing this ritual of balance and eating at least five balanced meals per day, you may also bring a more profound sense of balance into your daily life.

THE BASICS

Hot Point Nutrition is not a "diet," it is a way of eating. There are two ways of eating that will be discussed in this chapter. Truly, these two methods are simply two explanations of the same process. The first is quite easy to understand and even easier to implement and incorporate into your daily life. The first method, HOT POINT NUTRITION, is a very simple way to tailor your eating habits to fit your goals. The second method, EATING TO WIN, is virtually the same program, except that it becomes very exacting, taking in the precise number of calories you need to achieve your goals. When I think about "diet," I tend to look at it in much the same way I think of resistance training. After you learn the basics, you can refine and hone your technique forever. It is an endless process of performing the exercises to perfection. EATING TO WIN is very similar in that you are making your intake of food fit your goals to the exact calorie. Whether you subscribe to HOT POINT NUTRITION or EATING TO WIN, creating a sound nutritional program can and should be one of the easiest tasks you have ever performed. The trick is to get yourself into a habit of eating well.

Strange as it may seem, eating well means having at least five small and balanced meals per day, to keep the metabolism even, and not allowing your body to shift into a starvation mode. Eating well also means eating within 30 minutes of waking up in the morning, so your metabolism can begin working immediately. This program is all about creating positive habits, and this portion of the program is the easiest to understand, but it often requires the greatest mental discipline to master. If you can follow the Hot Point Nutrition program for two solid weeks, you will begin to lose the craving for foods that take you away from your goals, and begin craving and seeking out foods that take you toward your goals.

The idea here is to form a way of eating that you can adhere to for the rest of your life. Hot Point Nutrition could not be any easier. From this point forward, I want you to picture your meals as if there were two compartments on your plate. From now on, all of your meals will be based upon the ratio of protein to carbohydrates. Proteins and carbohydrates will always be eaten together in the same meal. A third dietary component, fat, does not get a compartment on your plate from this moment forward. Whatever fat is already in the food, and however much fat the food was cooked in, usually will be sufficient for your body to function normally.

Proteins and Carbohydrates

After you eat, the food must be digested. During the digestive process, the molecular structure of the food is broken down into smaller and smaller bits until these bits are small enough to pass through the intestinal wall and be released into the bloodstream. Once set free into the bloodstream, they can be used by the parts of the body that need them most. What your body ultimately derives from eating protein are amino acids. Amino acids feed lean muscle. The less fatty the protein, the more efficiently your lean muscle can utilize the amino acids. When carbohydrates are digested, they are ultimately broken down into glucose. You do need a certain amount of glucose to keep the body functioning properly, but when there is too much glucose in the bloodstream, it will cause a hormone called insulin to be secreted. Insulin has one job: to take out all the extra glucose in the bloodstream and store it within the fat cell just in case it is needed some time in the future. The problem is that once it is stored away, the body is very reluctant to part with it. It is therefore your primary objective not to flood the bloodstream with too much glucose. When choosing a carbohydrate, you will want to eat something that takes a long period of time to break apart in the digestive process, and you will find these listed in the diet as "Primary Carbohydrate Selections." Because the molecular chain of these particular carbohydrates is difficult to break apart, and because they do not pull apart easily, glucose is released into the bloodstream slowly and over a longer period of time. The more difficulty the body has in breaking apart the molecular chain of the carbohydrate, the higher the carbohydrate will appear on the list. I am certain you know what fat is. Fat is butter, oil, lard. . . the stuff that hangs over your belt . . . the stuff you want less of. Fat is essential for the body, and is essential in your diet. However, every living organism on the planet contains some fat, so it is not necessary to add any extra fat to your food. When cooking you should try to eliminate most, if not all, of the fat you can. Unfortunately, fat does add to the taste of food, so if you are going to add it, add it by the drop and not by the spoonful or cupful.

For any given meal, you should first decide which source of protein you will be eating, and then determine the carbohydrate choice and corresponding portion size. If you want to rid yourself of fat, the portion size of your protein should be approximately the size of your palm. If you want to maintain your present weight, your protein portion should be the size of your palm and the first joint of your finger. If you would like to gain muscle mass, your protein portion should be the size of your hand. In the diet, you will find a food list outlining which protein choices are best. There are good proteins and not-so-good proteins. A good protein would be the whey protein found in protein powder, egg whites, most fish, chicken breast, or turkey breast. These proteins have little inherent fat and are absorbed most effectively by your body's digestive system. A secondary, or not-so-good choice, would be choice cuts of beef that are highly marbled, pork products, sausages, processed meats, cold cuts, duck, goose, lamb, and cheese. All of these secondary choices contain a higher proportion of fat and are not absorbed effectively by your digestive system. More and more frequently, you should choose to cut these secondary choices out of your nutritional program.

Based on your choice of protein, you will determine which carbohydrate, and how much of that carbohydrate and fat, you should have. The size of your carbohydrate portion will be an exact ratio of either 1 to 1, or 1 to 2, the amount of protein on your plate. For instance, if you chose to eat one item from the list of "Primary Protein Selections," you could have twice that amount from the list of "Primary Carbohydrate Selections," or the exact same size portion of "Secondary

Carbohydrate Selections." In other words, if you were eating a skinless chicken breast, you could have twice the amount of steamed cauliflower (a 1-to-2 ratio), or the same size portion of rice, potato, bread, or pasta (a 1-to-1 ratio). If you chose to eat a secondary source of protein, you could have the same amount of a good carbohydrate or half that amount of a secondary carbohydrate selection. In other words, if you chose to eat a fatty protein like beef pot roast, you could eat that same portion size of steamed vegetables or half the portion size of your protein in pasta. In addition, there are a number of "free foods" that do not count toward the equation, and you may have as much of them as you like if you are still hungry.

There are a number of ways that you can play with the 1:1/1:2 model. If you chose an excellent protein source and were craving a piece of bread, you could fit it into your meal in the following way. Look at the portion of protein on your plate. Divide that surface area in half. That will be the portion of your bread. You can have the same-size portion of primary carbohydrates, and you will have completed the 1:2 meal. I know it is really more like the 1:1 1/2 meal, but you got the bread and you didn't make yourself crazy. Still hungry? A small tossed salad is a "Free Food," it does not count, and is not part of the equation unless you have croutons in your salad, or add any dressing other than vinegar, lemon, or a little salsa. So you might have had a chicken breast, some vegetables, a little bread, and a salad. That is really a nice meal, and you wouldn't feel like you were suffering if you did this five times a day, would you? What happens when you choose a secondary protein? Simply have the same-size portion of primary carbohydrates, or half that protein portion size of a secondary carbohydrate choice. Easy, right?

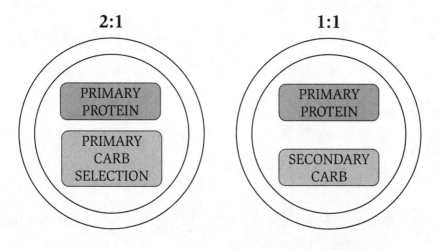

PRIMARY PROTEIN SELECTION

Chicken Breast (not processed)
Turkey Breast (not processed)
Lean Ground Beef (15% fat or lower)
Fish (any)
Shell Fish (any)
Fat-Free cheese
Egg Whites
Egg Substitutes
Cottage Cheese (low- or nonfat)
Protein Powder (whey)
Tofu
Soy Burger
Soy Hot Dog
Soy Sausages
ALL OTHERS = SECONDARY PROTEIN SELECTION

PRIMARY CARBOHYDRATE SELECTION

Vegetables

Artichoke
Asparagus
Dried Beans (any)
Green Beans
Soy Beans
Butter Beans
Bok Choy
Broccoli
Brussels Sprouts
Cabbage
Cauliflower
Chick peas
Eggplant
Kale

Kidney Beans
Red Beans
Lentils
Lima Beans
Mushrooms
Navy Beans
Pinto Beans
Spinach
Zucchini

Starchy Carbohydrates

Kellogg's Bran Bud with psyllium
Oatmeal (cooked)
Egg Noodles
Squash
Yams

Fruits

Apple
Cherries
Grapefruit
Peach
Pear
Plum
Strawberries

Yogurt

Non-fat with fruit & sugar substitute
Non-fat plain with sugar substitute
Non-fat, fruit-flavored with sugar

SECONDARY CARBOHYDRATE SELECTION

Breads (all)
Potatoes (all)
Most Rice
Most Cereals
Most Pasta
Beets
Carrots
Corn
Peas
Applesauce
Banana
Cantaloupe
Watermelon

Cranberries
Dates
Figs
Kiwi
Honeydew
Kumquats
Mango
Papaya
Prunes
Raisins
Tomato

Free Foods

Sugar-Free Instant Cocoa
Sugar-Free Sodas
Sugar-Free Jell-O
Crystal Light
Sugar-Free Iced Tea
Vinegar
Lime Juice
Lemon Juice
Mustard
Salsa
Garlic
Celery
Radishes
Peppers
Lettuce (iceberg, romaine, butter
    lettuce, endive, radicchio)

Jicama
Cucumber
Khalorabi

Before you begin your new nutritional program, here are a few helpful hints. Just to recap, you should have at least five small meals per day and be eating about every three hours. Have your normal breakfast, lunch, and dinner, and between these main meals have a snack consisting of a protein bar or shake, non-fat cottage cheese and fruit, or even a chicken breast with some raw vegetables. When eating, choose your protein first, and then choose the appropriate carbohydrate choice.

If you go out to eat, immediately order a tossed salad with dressing on the side. The point here is to avoid the breadbasket that will be placed on the table. My experience is that people dig into this bread as a matter of habit without fully realizing the amount of carbohydrates they are ingesting. I attempt to refrain from alcohol, but if you really need a glass of wine or a mixed drink, go ahead. If you have one drink, and I do mean ONE glass, this will count as your carbohydrate for the meal. Your meal could consist of a large dinner salad with lemon, a nice cut of beef or chicken breast, *and* a glass of wine.

Occasionally you will have cravings. You should choose one meal each week where you can eat whatever you like. Limit this to one meal per week and all should be well. If you want seven or eight of these meals in one week, chances are you will not see any results. Hot Point Nutrition takes some discipline, but after only a couple of weeks it will become second nature. Give yourself the gift of eating properly for those two weeks. It is a great chance, take it.

Drink a lot of water. You should have a minimum of 8 glasses of water a day. As ridiculous as it may sound, I would prefer if you drank at least a half-gallon. The body operates much better when you are hydrated. This is vital. You are almost 2/3 water, so it only makes sense that you need to replenish as much as possible. In addition to being essential, water is also one of the best ways to rid yourself of fat. Start with 8 glasses a day. Work your way up to a half-gallon. Once you can do this, try to work your way up to a gallon a day. If there is any color when you urinate, you aren't drinking enough.

Begin to keep a journal. If you have a day planner, or electronic wizard, jot down what you ate, when you ate, and how many glasses of water you drank during the day. This practice will help you in your discipline and may help you to make changes to your program as you begin to refine it. For some reason, when people begin to keep track of what they eat, they are better able to stick with their program.

The last hint that I have is to plan ahead. Eliminate all junk food from your house. Make certain that you have enough groceries on hand so that you do not order a pizza or go to the hamburger drive-thru out of desperation. Know what you are going to be eating. Plan your meals each day. If you work in an office, keep food in the fridge. Have some protein bars in your desk. Know which restaurants in your area serve or deliver the kind of food that you need.

Above all, this way of eating should not involve depriving yourself and should fit into your life reasonably. No one should eat less than 1,000 calories per day or the body will shift into a starvation mode, making it impossible for the body to shed body fat.

EATING TO WIN

There are some people who are not following any certain diet or nutritional plan. For them, following the Hot Point Nutrition program would be a breakthrough in itself, and there is no doubt that they would come closer to realizing their dreams and reaching their goals. But for some people to get results, they must really reign in their nutritional program and make it exact. Most of my celebrity and pro-athlete clients are so focused on and dedicated to their fitness program that they actually need a strict eating regimen. Some other clients are so motivated to attain their goals that they want to do anything and everything in their power to realize their goals. Some people just simply do not get the results they are looking for when they approach their nutritional program in a casual manner and need to make their diets more exact. If you are in a similar position, here is all the information you'll need to create a nutritional program that is absolutely perfect for you. Where the first half of this chapter was quite simple to follow and had a fairly loose guideline, Eating To Win is fairly complex, requiring you to be extremely dedicated, and to measure your food and count your caloric intake for each meal.

EATING TO WIN will use a different model to determine what you should eat for each meal. This model is based upon calories. For this program, 40% of your calories should be derived from protein, 40% should be derived from carbohydrates, and 20% of your calories should be derived from fat. To determine what and how much you should eat, get out your body-fat measurements and your calculator.

To determine what and how much you should be eating, you will first need to determine what your total caloric intake should be per day. This requires some calculation, so for the moment just fill in the blanks, as I walk you through the equation.

The first numbers you want to determine are your weight, your body-fat percentage, the number of pounds you have in fat, and the amount of your total weight that is lean muscle mass. Ready to start? Let's begin with the easiest number to determine.

Your weight on the scale _____

Multiply your weight by your body-fat percentage
(place the decimal point in front of this number)

weight _____ x . _____ body-fat percentage = _____ pounds of fat
This is the total number of pounds of fat that you have.

(It's only math—keep going!)

Subtract your weight on the scale from the number of pounds of fat
pounds of fat _____ – _____ weight on scale = _____ your lean muscle mass.

This is a very important number. Lumped into this number is not only muscle, but your bones, your organs, your hair and nails. This is what we want to feed. Your lean muscle mass requires protein for fuel. The amount of protein you actually need will depend upon your activity level. If you are in Phase One, you need 1 gram of protein per pound of lean muscle mass. If you are in Phase Two, you need 1.25 grams of protein per pound of lean muscle mass. If you are in Phase Three, you will need 1.5 grams of protein per pound of lean muscle mass.

DETERMINE HOW MANY GRAMS OF PROTEIN YOU NEED EACH DAY

Phase One Lean Muscle Mass _____ x 1.00 = _____ Grams of protein per day
Phase Two Lean Muscle Mass _____ x 1.25 = _____ Grams of protein per day
Phase Three Lean Muscle Mass _____ x 1.50 = _____ Grams of protein per day

How much protein should I have with each meal?

Would you prefer to eat five times per day or six times per day? _____
Divide the grams of protein you need _____ ÷ _____ number of meals = _____
This is the number of grams of protein you should have with each meal.

How many calories should I have each day?

Grams of protein I need per meal _____ x 4 (calories in one gram of protein) =
_____. This is the amount of calories you need to derive from protein each time
you eat.

*Multiply this number by two, because you will want the same number of calories
from carbohydrates.*

Protein calories _____ x 2 = _____. This is the total number of calories from proteins and carbohydrates, which leaves fat.

Carry over the last number, and divide that number by .8 (fat calories).

Calories from protein and carbs _____ ÷ .8 = _____ (calories per meal).

Multiply calories per meal by the number of meals you would like to eat each day.

Calories per meal_____ x _____ (5 or 6 meals) = _____.

This is the total number of calories you want to ingest every day.

I NEED TO EAT EXACTLY _____ CALORIES PER DAY.

You now know what and how much you need to be eating, how many times per
day you should be eating, how many calories you should have with each meal, and
best of all, you just saved yourself hundreds of dollars in nutritionist's bills. You
have now determined exactly how many calories you need to take in each day to
make your nutritional program work to perfection. Counting calories may not be the
most exciting task that you have ever performed in your life, but it will mean getting
the results you are looking for. Most of the packaged foods that you will find at the
grocery store will have this information on the label. However, when you go shopping, are cooking at home, and when you go out to eat at a restaurant, you will need
to become familiar with the caloric value of the foods that you eat to stay within
your program. At the end of this chapter, I have provided a list of foods with a cor-

responding caloric value. While this is by no means a complete list of all the foods that exist, the list does represent the foods that would be primary meal choices. If you find that many of the foods you eat are not on this list, you should either consider changing your eating habits slightly or pick up one of the many pocket books that offer a complete list of the caloric value of food.

The first two rules of EATING TO WIN are 1) never have less than 1,000 calories per day or your body will go into a starvation mode; and 2) never have more than 50 grams of protein in one sitting. Unfortunately, this ruins the equation for some of you. If you have under 100 pounds of lean muscle mass and you are in Phase Two, or if you have over 200 pounds of lean muscle mass and are in Phase Three, you will need to make some adjustments. If you do not fit into either of these categories, please skip ahead to the next paragraph. If you have under 100 pounds of lean muscle mass and you are in Phase Two, you will need to make the following adjustments so that your total caloric intake exceeds 1000 calories. Simply add another meal so that you are eating seven meals per day, instead of six. You will need this extra meal to maintain your lean muscle mass and the proper functioning of your vital organs. This should bring you above 1000 calories, and should prevent your body from shifting into a starvation mode and thereby not allowing your body to burn fat to fuel your activity. If you have over 200 pounds of lean muscle mass and you are in Phase Three, you will also need to make a slight adjustment so that you are not consuming over 50 grams of protein per meal. Simply take your total caloric intake and add an extra meal so that you are now eating seven meals per day instead of six. Your body needs the protein to be spread out more evenly throughout the day for you to get the results you are looking for.

In order for this program to work at the highest possible level, your body needs water to process the foods appropriately. Drinking at least a half-gallon of water a day will not only help you digest the food more efficiently, it will help you to purge body fat out of your system. Because you are physically active, this water intake can be increased almost infinitely to maintain the hydration level, keep your hair and skin looking great, and make you less hungry.

Whereas the strategy in Hot Point Weight Training is to shock the body to get the desired result, the strategy for eating is the exact opposite. To disarm the starvation protection system in your body, you need to eat at least five small balanced meals per day. Try your hardest to eat at almost exactly the same times each day for the first two weeks. Your body will soon assimilate to this schedule and trust that it will be fed regularly. The more regular your eating schedule, the less likely your body will be to fear that it will starve, and therefore be more certain that it can expend the stored energy within the fat cells to fuel your activity. Because you will need to be feeding yourself every two-and-a-half to three hours, you will need to plan ahead to keep yourself on track. If you know you will be away from your home or your office for an extended period of time, bring enough food with you so that you do not fall off the wagon. By eating frequently, you are raising your metabolism to burn hot and fast. Take a lesson from children. They seem to be almost constantly eating, and yet most are not particularly fat. Yes, they are growing, but so are you. Each time you work out you are increasing the density in your lean muscle. When you miss a meal, your metabolism is allowed to slow down. At this stage the most harmful things you can do are to not eat, and when you do eat, to overeat, making up for the meal or meals that you missed. Invariably, you will lose any momentum you gained and end up putting body fat back on very quickly.

For the first two weeks you are on this program, I suggest that you weigh and measure almost everything that you eat. Soon you will know by sight what something weighs, or in the case of liquids, know how much volume it has, and you will have reasonable certainty of your caloric intake when you go out to eat at a restaurant.

As with the more casual Hot Point Nutrition, you should keep a daily journal and make note of everything you put in your mouth and what time you ate. I know that this may sound a little obsessive, but in keeping a journal, you will automatically become more regular and consistent in your feeding pattern. You will also help yourself to stay within the caloric boundaries of your nutritional program. With all that said, you should take a look at where and how you will fulfill your nutritional program in terms of the calories that you will take in. Here is a list of foods with their corresponding caloric value.

	Portion	Protein	Carbs	Fat	Calories
Chicken breast	1 oz.	6	0	Trace	30
Turkey breast	1 oz.	7	0	Trace	28
Ground beef – 15% or less	3 oz.	22	0	14	217
All fish					
Fat-free cheese					
Egg whites	1	4	Trace	0	17
Egg substitute	1/4 cup	6	1	0	25
Cottage cheese lowfat	1 cup	28	6	2	164
Cottage cheese nonfat	4.4 oz.	15	7	0	90
Apple	1	Trace	21	Trace	81
Cherries	1 cup	1	19	1	90
Grapefruit	1/2	1	14	0	50
Peach	1	1	10	Trace	37
Pear	1	1	25	1	98
Plum	1	1	9	Trace	36
Whole wheat spaghetti	2 oz.	8	43	Trace	198
Fettucini	2.5 oz.	7	39	2	190
Vermicelli	2 oz.	9	40	1	210
Artichoke	1 med. (4 oz.)	4	13	Trace	60
Asparagus	4 spears	2	3	Trace	14
Black beans	1/2 cup	9	19	1	90
Green beans	1/2 cup	1	4	0	16
Navy beans	1/2 cup (4.5 oz.)	6	19	1	110
Soy beans	1/2 cup	11	10	6	127
Butter beans	1/2 cup(4.5 oz.)	7	22	1	120
Peas	1/2 cup	4	12	1	60
Baked beans	1/2 cup	6	26	1	118
Bok choy	1/2 cup	1	0	4	136
Broccoli	1/2 cup	2	4	Trace	22
Brussel sprouts	1/2 cup	2	7	Trace	30

(continues)

	Portion	Protein	Carbs	Fat	Calories
Cabbage	1/2 cup (2.6 oz.)	1	3	Trace	17
Cauliflower	1/2 cup (2.2 oz.)	1	3	Trace	14
Chick peas	1 cup	12	54	3	285
Egg plant	1/2 cup	Trace	3	Trace	13
Kale	1/2 cup	1	4	Trace	21
Kidney beans	1 cup	13	38	1	208
Lentils	1 cup	18	40	1	231
Lima beans	1/2 cup	6	18	Trace	94
Mushrooms	1 (1/2 oz.)	Trace	1	Trace	5
Onions	1/2 cup	1	5	Trace	21
Spinach	3 oz.	3	Trace	Trace	9
Yellow squash	1/2 cup (4.2 oz.)	0	5	0	25
Pinto beans	1/2 cup	6	20	0	100
Zucchini	1/2 cup	1	4	Trace	14
Yogurt (plain, nonfat)	8 oz.	13	17	Trace	127
Potato	1 (6 1/2 oz.)	5	51	Trace	220
Rice	1/2 cup	3	23	Trace	109
Apple sauce	1/2 cup	Trace	14	Trace	53
Banana	1	1	27	Trace	105
Cantaloupe (cubed)	1 cup	1	13	Trace	57
Cranberries	1/2 cup	Trace	54	Trace	209
Dates	10	2	61	Trace	228
Figs (fresh)	1 med.	Trace	10	Trace	50
Kiwi	1 med.	1	11	Trace	46
Honeydew melon (cubed)	1 cup	1	16	Trace	60
Kumquats	1	Trace	3	Trace	12
Mango	1	1	35	1	135
Papaya (cubed)	1 cup	1	30	Trace	54
Prunes (pitted)	1/4 cup (1.4 oz.)	1	29	0	120
Raisins	1.5 oz.	0	33	0	140
Beets	1/2 cup	1	22	Trace	89
Carrots	1 (1/2 oz.)	Trace	1	Trace	6

	Portion	Protein	Carbs	Fat	Calories
Yam (cubed)	1/2 cup	1	19	Trace	79
Red Vinegar	1 oz.	0	0	0	4
Celery	1 stalk (1.3 oz.)	Trace	1	Trace	6
Lettuce (Romaine)	1-1/2 cups	1	2	1	18
Egg Fetuccini	2 oz.	10	38	3	210
Kellogg's Bran Bud	1/3 cup (1 oz.)	3	24	0	70
Oatmeal (cooked)	1/2 cup	5	27	3	150

6

Burn Fat at a White Hot Pace

Hot Point Aerobics

The great catalyst for Hot Point Fitness, and the most addictive and self-gratifying element of the program, is aerobic activity. Aerobic activity forms the groundwork for the program, and with resistance training and nutrition completes the three sides of the Hot Point pyramid. With Hot Point Fitness, you will be using resistance training to tone, define, and create density throughout your muscles. Hot Point Nutrition promotes the creation and growth of lean muscle mass and discourages and prevents the build-up of stored fat. Hot Point Aerobics eliminates excess body fat and increases your level of fitness, endurance, and promotes your overall health. Where weight training represents the means to achieve your physical transformation, that physical transformation can only take place with the support of a sound nutritional program coupled with regular aerobic activity. While Hot Point Resistance Training is presented to you in a structured manner, you need to create your own diet based upon your individual needs and also create your own complimentary aerobic exercise program. Like the previous chapter on nutrition, Hot Point Aerobics will serve as a guideline so you can create the program that best suits your needs, and the program that will bring you toward your goal quickly, safely, and efficiently.

Why Should I Do Aerobics?

There are so many questions and so much confusion surrounding aerobic exercise that it is best to get these answers up front. When I talk about aerobics to people who are new to exercise, they usually conjure up 1980s images of celebrities in leotards and headbands. While discussing the topic of aerobics, I am not necessarily referring to a class with 50 sweating people moving to a pulsing beat. Aerobic exercise takes many forms. The biggest question is, "Why should I do it?" The answer is simple. You will improve your health, and you will burn off calories. Regular aerobic exercise will strengthen your heart, improve your circulation, flush your system of toxins, offset major aging issues like osteoporosis, and also boost your immune system. In addition to adding to your health and longevity, there is no better way to reduce the layer of fat underneath your skin.

Hot Point Aerobics is geared to heat your muscles, increase your metabolism, and burn off calories like they were on fire. In terms of your transformation, the point is to have a greater and greater level of fitness and stamina. However, the true importance of aerobics, within the context Hot Point Fitness, is to speed your metabolism. The more fit you become, the more calories your body will burn when you are at rest. A better-trained individual will burn 20% more calories at rest than a sedentary person does.

There are many attributes and even more long-term health benefits associated with regular aerobic exercise. Aerobic exercise can decrease your appetite. Exercising within your ideal target range allows for greater caloric intake without gaining fat. Aerobic exercise has been scientifically proven to strengthen the skeletal system, creating bone density and combating osteoporosis. This form of exercise is most often a part of the treatment for diabetics, those recovering from heart attacks, those counteracting high blood pressure, and those on a program to lower cholesterol. In addition to reducing the risk of coronary artery disease, regular aerobic exercise helps those suffering from arthritis. Perhaps the greatest benefit is that aerobically fit people deal with stress much more effectively. Although it is not documented, I feel that in this day and age, stress might be the number one health risk in our society, and aerobic activity is certainly a proven and effective tool to combat that stress.

For most people, the point is to get your body hot. Literally and figuratively, this means warming your muscles up, supercharging the metabolism to burn off excess calories, and elevating your heart rate to a certain level for a certain period of time to melt the fat off of your body. When you can do this regularly and consistently, you will call upon stored fat to fuel your activity. You will burn up your caloric intake. And soon you will look absolutely HOT.

Aerobic & Anaerobic Exercise

When you exercise, you burn calories to fuel your activity. The point of Hot Point Aerobics is to burn those calories off in the most efficient manner possible. There are two levels of exercise and consequently two ways that you can burn off calories: one is anaerobic, the other is called aerobic. Both of these terms refer to the manner in which the calorie is utilized or "burned" by your body. When you exercise and elevate your heart rate significantly, blood is passed through the muscles being worked. To fuel that activity, the muscle extracts its fuel from the blood cell. When you are exercising at 50% to 80% of your maximum heart rate, glucose is extracted from the blood cell. At this level of exercise, you are in an aerobic state. When your heart rate reaches 85% to 100% of its maximum, there is so much blood pumping through your system that your body does not have enough time to process it all. To get around this dilemma, it simply burns the cell wall, or mitochondria, to fuel the activity. When this occurs, you are in an anaerobic state. You can exercise at an aerobic level for a very long time. However, when you reach an anaerobic level, you can only sustain it for a few seconds before you either have to stop or slow down. If you were running a 100-yard dash, you might be at an aerobic state for the first three or four seconds of the race. If you really kicked it into high gear and pushed yourself to your physical limit, you would achieve an anaerobic state for only the last six seconds of the race. When you are in an anaerobic state, you are truly exhausting the energy supply because you are burning through the blood cells at such a rapid rate. The mitochondria cannot provide the muscles with the pure energy they need to keep going. After reaching the anaerobic state for a maximum duration of five to ten seconds, the body just shuts down, and you will be forced to either slow down or stop altogether. You may have seen examples of this if you have ever watched Olympic runners or seen a horse race. Some of the participants may have peaked too early in the race, and at the end of the race they appear to be slowing down rather than accelerating towards the finish line. Another example of this would be weight lifting. As you will soon experience, you will be asking yourself to perform three sets of a specific weight lifting exercise. Each of these sets is made up of several repetitions. You will be at an aerobic level for the great majority of the set, but during the last three or four repetitions, you will begin to feel a sense of fatigue. You will have to struggle to push the weight until you reach a point of muscular failure and are no longer physically able to perform another repetition. You will have reached the anaerobic phase of the exercise, and your body will force you to stop.

With Hot Point Aerobics, you will consciously manipulate the aerobic and anaerobic states to meet your goals. The program is very simple to follow and is easy to incorporate into your lifestyle. During your workout, you will begin with five minutes of aerobics to warm up the muscles in your body. By stretching between resistance exercises, you will remain in an aerobic state throughout your workout, reaching anaerobic levels toward the end of each set. To end your workout, you will perform at least 25 minutes of the aerobic activity of your own choosing and consciously reach anaerobic levels several times during each session.

Getting Aerobic

To reach an aerobic level that burns fat, you will need to elevate your heart rate. Your body will burn calories most efficiently when your heart rate is between 60% and 80% of the maximum heart rate. There is an equation that determines what your maximum heart rate is. Let me walk you through this equation so that you can determine where your most efficient levels are. You may want a calculator to determine these numbers. And you should write these numbers down so that you can refer to them later.

Your heart should never beat more that 220 times per minute. The medical establishment has created this ceiling, and if your heart rate exceeds it, you enter a danger zone of sorts. At all costs, you should never surpass this magic number. With the maximum of 220 beats per minute, simply subtract your age from that number. For instance, if you are 40 years old, your maximum heart rate would be 180 (220–40 = 180).

This number will be your personal ceiling. I repeat, you never want to go above this number. When you are performing the aerobic portion of this program, you will want to maintain your heart rate in the 60% – 80% range for the majority of your session. So let's determine what that means in terms of your personal target area. Using our example of the person who is 40 years of age, they would multiply 180 x .60 and then multiply 180 x .80. The ideal aerobic level for a 40-year-old would be when the heart beats between 108 and 144 times per minute.

Do one last calculation to determine where you reach your anaerobic state. Remember, when you reach this threshold you can only sustain it for a very brief spurt of energy. You will be entering into this range for a brief period of time and do so consciously only to achieve a desired result. The anaerobic state is reached when you achieve 90% of your maximum heart rate. Again using the 40-year-old as an example, the number would be determined by multiplying the maximum heart rate of 180 by .90. (180 x .90 = 162). When their heart reaches 162 beats per minute, they will only be able to sustain that activity for a maximum of ten seconds, and then they will either have to slow way down or stop altogether.

Monitoring Your Heart Rate

Now that you have calculated your ideal heart rate, you need to know how to find your pulse. There are three methods to determine how many times per minute your heart is beating. Two of these methods can be done manually with the aid of a clock or stopwatch, and the other is by utilizing a small machine. You can take your own pulse on two points of the body—one at the wrist and the other on the neck. Finding these spots takes a little practice, but after you have identified them and become familiar with them, they will prove to be fairly decent indicators of your heart rate. The point on the wrist is sometimes easier to find. Find the point at which your forearm meets the hand. Place your pointing and middle fingers in the middle of that area. (Never use your thumb as this finger has its own pulse.) You will feel a tendon or even several tendons in your wrist. Move your fingers slowly to the inside portion of your wrist until you can find the pulse at its strongest point. The other point at which you can accurately measure your pulse is in the neck, or the carotid artery. To find this artery, locate the point where the front of your neck muscles meet your throat. Move your fingers slowly up the inside neck muscle until you find the point at which the pulse is the strongest. With your fingers on either of these two spots, refer to a clock that has a second hand or to a stopwatch. Count the number of heartbeats for fifteen seconds. Multiply that number by four and you have successfully determined your heart rate. If this gets too complicated or cumbersome, there is a third option.

There are a number of heart monitors on the market that do this for you. I personally prefer these devices over taking my own pulse, as they are more accurate and I find looking at a monitor to be less of a hassle. These heart monitors are small and inconspicuous and are usually attached to a belt or elastic strap. The belt is placed around your chest and acts as a monitor. The monitor relays information to a watch worn on your wrist. While you are exercising, you only have to look at your wristwatch and you can check your levels instantly.

The reason we want to monitor our heart rate is threefold. The first reason is simple. Studies have proven that people who exercise at 60% – 80% of their maximum heart rate levels are much more likely to exercise regularly. If you have ever attempted regular exercise and have just stopped for no apparent reason, you may have been exercising at a rate that your body could not sustain. It is far more taxing for your body to operate at 85% of your maximum. And if you do so over an extended period of time, you may get burned out and quit exercising altogether. The second consideration is time. As always, you want to make this program time-efficient, or to get the greatest result in the quickest possible manner. Thirdly, exercising at 60% – 80% of your maximum heart rate is the exact level at which the body burns calories at the most efficient level possible.

How Long Should I Exercise?

When you are exercising aerobically, you need to keep your heart rate in the 60%–80% range for at least 25 minutes to have the desired result. When you are in your ideal aerobic range for this length of time, you will burn calories at the most efficient rate possible. For the first ten minutes or so, the body will use the glucose within the blood stream to fuel the motion. In other words, you will be expending the excess calories you have eaten. For the next 15 minutes, the bloodstream will not be able to provide the body with all its needed fuel, so it will have to call upon its reserve tank, or stored fat, to provide the necessary energy. In these all-important 15 minutes, you will be fueling your activity with 50% from the glucose that still is in the bloodstream. The other 50% of the expended calories will be derived from burning up the fat that is stored underneath your skin. If you can stay nearer to 80% of your maximum heart rate throughout your workout, you can call upon an even greater percentage of stored fat. If your goal is to rid yourself of body fat more quickly, you may want to devote more time to your aerobic workout. You could exercise aerobically for several hours, but the truth of the matter is that after 60 minutes or so, you will have maximized your workout. My recommendation is to do at least 25 minutes of aerobic exercise and no more than one hour, unless you are consciously performing extra aerobic activity to achieve a specific fitness goal.

How Often Should I Do Aerobics?

You must perform this aerobic workout at least three times per week, and can safely do this as many as six days per week. As with all forms of exercise, you must take at least one day off per week to let the body rest, heal, and recuperate. It is best to space out the days of your aerobic exercise to get the greatest result. Instead of performing your workouts on three consecutive days and resting for four, you should space the workouts evenly throughout the week. In so doing, you will boost your metabolism, burn calories more efficiently, and ultimately have greater success.

Surprise, Surprise, Surprise

The last point I would like to stress to you about aerobic exercise is perhaps the most important. The single most vital ingredient to maximizing your aerobic workout is to vary your workout. The body is very reluctant to rid itself of body fat, and you must outthink it consistently. The body is resilient and will conserve its fuel whenever it can, so you must trick it. If you do the exact same aerobic exercise each and every time you work out, after only a short while the body will give up less and less stored fat. To prevent this, you will want to vary the way in which you work out. If you are on the treadmill, you may want to increase or decrease the incline level every other time you work out. If you are jogging, you may not want to just run around the track at the exact same pace; you may want to do bursts when you elevate the heart rate to 85% and bring it back down to the ideal range, and then vary how long those bursts last. Better yet, you may want to get off the track and jog through different areas, and each day find an area with a differing terrain. Many of the machines I will talk about in the paragraphs to come have different courses that simulate this exact principle. You should make a note of which course you did last and be certain to change it around for the next workout. You may choose to perform completely different exercises on different days. By employing some or all of these strategies, you will keep your body in a state of surprise. In this way, you can keep your body guessing and always demand the maximum result for your efforts.

The Hot Point Performance Zone

By varying your routine, and always increasing and decreasing the level of difficulty while you exercise, you also push yourself to become more physically fit. As you become more fit, your aerobic ceiling will increase. This is what you are striving for. Instead of becoming fatigued when you exercise at 60% of your maximum heart rate, you may have to increase to 70% or 80% as you grow stronger. In other words, it will take more effort to shift into an anaerobic gear. You can increase your performance envelope by practicing terrain variance. If, during your aerobic workout, you were to jog in a hilly terrain or have the computerized resistance level on the treadmill set to vary the incline level you were jogging on, there would be times when you achieved an anaerobic level of exercise. As you near the top of the hill, your body is working harder. As a result, your heart rate increases to a point at which you may reach anaerobic levels of exercise. Typically, the signals that you have reached this anaerobic stage will include a shortness of breath, lactic acid buildup, and the onset of rapid fatigue. When you can facilitate brief encounters with the anaerobic stage and come back into your target area of 60% to 80%, you will successfully improve your physical condition, eliminate much of the glucose in the bloodstream, and consequently burn a greater number of calories from stored fat when you return to your targeted aerobic range.

Just Do It!

There are many different ways to achieve an aerobic level and there are no excuses for avoiding this important element of your transformation. If you have a tendency to avoid aerobic exercise like the plague, I again ask you to re-commit yourself to the process. You cannot get to the destination you want by avoiding this. Challenge and push yourself just to show up. Promise yourself that you will do ten minutes. After those first ten minutes are up, you are less likely to give up on yourself. During those first minutes, try to visualize your goal. Whatever your goal, your transformation depends heavily on doing your aerobic workout. You have a vast array of options, and there is no reason that you should ever become bored by your choices.

What Kind of Aerobics Should I Do?

I separate these activities into two categories: indoor and outdoor. Because of the friction involved in outdoor activities, you may actually burn more calories. But depending on the weather, you may choose to do either. There are a number of team sports that can be played outdoors: soccer, field hockey, and basketball. Many sports, such as racquetball, squash, and handball are fantastic indoor aerobic activities. However, you do not have to belong to a team, have a partner, or participate in an organized league to enjoy the benefits of aerobic exercise. I prefer individual activities, so that I do not have the excuse of "my partner didn't show up" for not getting in my aerobics. I also prefer to do my aerobic workout immediately after I finish my weight training. While lifting weights, there is an increased amount of lactic acid in the body. And completing the aerobic portion at this time may prevent a great deal of soreness, especially on the days when you work out your legs.

Outdoor

Some may like to jog; others may like to walk; some like swing-dancing; others enjoy non-impact activities like swimming; others still would prefer to ride their bicycle. It doesn't matter as long as you raise your heart rate to the ideal range and never, ever, stop until at least 25 minutes have passed. This means that if you choose to walk, it is not the kind of window shopping at the mall walk, but a brisk pace with energetic motion in the arms. You might choose to bring a set of two-pound dumbbells on your walk to increase the workout. You may live in a high-rise building and choose to walk the staircase from top to bottom. You may want to bring the jump rope outdoors and take in the sun while you do your aerobics. You may want to ride your bike through different parts of the city each day, varying terrain frequently enough so that your body does not become used to the workout. You may choose a nice swim. Swimming is perhaps the most beneficial choice, as through this activity you are truly working every muscle group in the body to elevate your heart rate and are using resistance and stretching techniques simultaneously with every stroke. This form of exercise also has an added advantage of not putting stress on the joints and limiting the possibility of injury.

Indoor

I strongly suggest that you do your aerobics as part of a total workout. You are already at the gym, so why not finish what you started. At the gym you will find many options to complete your aerobic exercise. Most gyms offer aerobics classes. These are not what they used to be. Rather than being the passé dance-like fashion show, they have gone through a significant evolution and have adapted many disciplines. There are now classes that stress high impact, low impact, jazzercise, hip-hop, country western, resistance aerobics, kick-boxing, aerobics using an elevated step, a form of aerobics that is performed on a stationary bike called spinning, and even water aerobics. In addition to being a lot of fun, these classes are supervised and are offered frequently enough so that it fits your schedule. In addition to the vast array of aerobics classes, there are many machines available for your purposes. Most gyms are equipped with stationary bikes, rowing machines, stair masters, ski machines, treadmills, the versiclimber, and a machine called an elliptical trainer. As you are left to your own supervision while using these devices, I would like to briefly discuss each of the machines and provide some ideas that can maximize results when you use them.

Rowing

The rowing machine is a fantastic method to achieve an aerobic workout. You are using many, if not all, of your body's muscle groups with this form of exercise. Although this is one of the most effective forms of aerobic exercise, it is the machine that is the least likely to sustain your interest for long-term usage. For the best results on this machine, you should vary the intensity of your rowing pace. You may begin at a relatively relaxed pace, to bring your heart rate up to the 60% range, and after a few minutes take it up to 70%. At the ten-minute mark, begin to perform your interval training. Do this by increasing your heart rate to 80% for two minutes and bring it back down to 70% for three minutes. Five minutes before the end of your exercise session, reduce your heart rate to 60% for the remainder of the exercise. Each day you exercise on the rowing machine, begin the interval training 30 seconds sooner. After only a short time, you will be starting your interval training at the one-minute mark. When you have reached this point, begin extending the intervals at which you achieve 85% of your maximum heart rate by 15 seconds, and decreasing by 15 seconds the portion of the interval where you are at 80% of your maximum heart rate.

Stationary Bike

The stationary bike is one of the most used machines at the gym, and in my opinion, one of the least effective at giving you a sufficient cardiovascular workout, primarily because the entire upper portion of your body is not in motion. When you are walking or jogging, rowing or skiing, the arms are swinging or moving. As a result, the heart must be called upon to pump blood to these limbs, increasing both your circulation and heart rate. If you choose to use the stationary bike, you should always create arm movement. Pump your arms, use one or two pound dumbbells for curls and an assortment of tricep exercises, or even try boxing-like motions with your arms to involve your upper body and increase your heart rate. If you do not involve your arms with some kind of motion, you will have to pedal furiously to get your heart rate up, and you may not finish your aerobic workout. If you do involve the arms with some kind of movement, it is best to select a random course setting where you can effectively raise and lower the intensity of resistance. The random course will simulate riding up and down an assortment of hills and ask you to increase and decrease the speed at which you do so. Most computerized stationary bikes have a number of course selections, and you should use a different course each time you exercise on this machine. If the stationary bike you are using does not have computerized controls, simply increase and decrease the resistance level in specific time intervals and change those intervals each time you exercise on that machine.

The Treadmill

The treadmill is an excellent machine to take you into your aerobic target zone. This machine is best utilized by **not** holding onto the handrails. Like the stationary bike, the machine is maximized when you can involve the upper half of your body. When you walk or jog on the treadmill and do not hold onto the handrails, your arms will naturally swing back and forth. Like many other aerobic machines at the gym, a computer will often control the treadmill you use. The computer controls will increase the incline level you are walking or jogging on to simulate the experience of going up and down hills. There are a number of courses to choose from, with a wide array of speeds. Make a note of what you did today and do a different course tomorrow.

The Stair Master

The step machine, otherwise known as the Stair Master, is another fine choice to give you an excellent aerobic workout. While some find this a difficult workout, it is actually my personal preference. Like the stationary bike and the treadmill, this machine is most effective when you can involve your arms. Most people who have used this machine complain that it not effective. Most people who use this machine also use it incorrectly because they hold onto the handrails and let their arms support most of their weight. Used correctly, these handrails should only give you balance. If you can avoid using the handrails altogether, this machine actually provides a challenging and invigorating aerobic workout. Where exercising on the treadmill will provide periods when you are walking or jogging over a flat terrain, the step machine always simulates the experience of going uphill. Choose a different computerized course each day to get the greatest results. Aside from providing a great sweat, this machine also can bring definition to the calves, the thighs, and gluteal (butt) muscles.

The Elliptical Trainer

The elliptical trainer is arguably the finest possible choice of gym equipment to meet your aerobic needs. The elliptical trainer uses the best attributes of all the machines previously mentioned and combines them all into one effective device. The footrests are designed to move in the shape of a football, and because of this design, the machine is termed low impact, reducing the risk of injury to the knees and joints. This machine is usually equipped with the most sophisticated computer, which regulates the incline level in an almost endless array of courses. Each course selection can be quite different, and ensures you will not become bored with frequent use. In essence, the elliptical trainer gives you the low-impact workout you would get on the stationary bike, simulates the walking or jogging motion that you would enjoy on the treadmill, and trains over a hilly terrain not unlike the Stair Master. In addition to providing a fantastic workout that eliminates the possibility of injury, the elliptical trainer also provides secondary benefits in terms of developing and defining the musculature in the thighs, calves, and buttocks. Like the stationary bike and Stair Master, you must consciously involve the arms when using this machine. The more movement in your arms, the greater the circulation. And, of course, the greater the circulation, the greater the health benefits associated with aerobic exercise.

Putting Together Your Aerobic Program

Before you begin the workouts that are outlined in the chapters to follow, it is important that you are able to complete at least 20 minutes of continuous aerobic activity. Please always keep in mind that you are not a failure if you cannot complete a 20-

minute session. It only means that you have to work up to this level before you begin Phase One of your workouts. If you are not used to regular exercise, you may want to begin slowly. Try starting with 5 minutes the first time out. Each time you exercise, increase the time you spend by 2 1/2 minutes, until get up to 20 minutes. While you are working your way up to this level, it is a good strategy to stay around 60% of your maximum heart rate. By working your way up slowly, and by not overexerting yourself, you will be able to get to the 20-minute mark more quickly and without becoming turned off to the notion of aerobic exercise. By the time you begin Phase One, you will find yourself looking forward to your aerobic sessions.

As you begin your workouts in Phase One, Phase Two, or Phase Three, you will note that at the end of each workout session there is a suggested time for you to engage in continuous aerobic activity. In Phase One, you will begin with 20 minutes and work your way up to 30 minutes as the program progresses. In Phase Two and Phase Three, your aerobic workout increases gradually and is designed in this way so not only are you becoming more fit throughout the program but you are also accelerating the rate at which you are shedding unwanted body fat. However, the recommended time I suggest for your aerobic workout may not always be in sync with your goals.

Hot Point Fitness can be adjusted slightly to better suit your needs. The number of minutes that are suggested at the end of each workout reflect the minimum amount of aerobic activity you need to achieve your goals. For instance, in Phase One you absolutely and positively need to engage in some form of aerobic activity for at least 20 minutes, three times per week. If your goal is to rid yourself of body fat more quickly, you may want to consider extending the number of minutes in the aerobic portion of your workout, or even adding an aerobic session on one of the days you are not working out. Again, the number of minutes suggested is the *minimum* amount of aerobics you need. Some of my clients do one hour of aerobics as soon as they wake up, and another hour of aerobics after they complete their workout. It is really up to you. Just remember that after about an hour or so, the fat-burning benefits taper off quickly, and also keep in mind that you need one full day of rest per week to let your body recuperate and heal.

Feeling Great

Even if you dread doing your aerobics, I promise that this will become the most addictive portion of your program. By doing your aerobics, not only are you potentially adding years to your life, but you are also gaining an abundance of health-related benefits that will give a heightened sense of quality to those years. You will notice a difference in the way your skin looks, the quality of your hair will improve, you will flush toxins from your system, and you will notice a significant difference in your energy level. Even more dramatic than your health, you will see a dramatic difference in the way you relate to others. While you are doing aerobics, endomorphins are released into your system. These endomorphins give you a mood-altering euphoric feeling and provide a joyful sense of well-being. By exercising regularly, you are much more capable of handling stressful situations coolly and calmly, and you will see that you are much more capable and productive at work, and have much more patience and quality time with the people who are closest to you. Combine this with shedding body fat and looking fantastic, and I believe that you have a recipe for the greatest and most positive addiction of all time.

PART 2

The Hot Point Workouts

7

Phase One—3 day a week workout routines

This is where the fun starts. This is the moment when your life changes. I know you are anxious to get started, but a word of caution before you begin . . . If you were overzealous and have skipped ahead to this chapter, I encourage you to go back and carefully read the previous chapters as doing so will speed your results immeasurably.

Because I am not at your side cheering you on, this book will be the conduit between us. Even if you have read the previous chapters, you may find it helpful to refer to them occasionally to refresh your memory or to improve upon your technique. Remember, there is no exercise that cannot be improved upon infinitely, and there are slight variations and wholly new exercises for you in this book. The goal of these exercises and philosophy are completely different than anything you have ever tried before. I will attempt to make this process very similar to the experience you would have if you had hired me to be your personal trainer. It is, therefore, vital that you bring your trainer to the gym with you in the form of this book.

Take careful measurements and note the particular areas of the body that might be out of balance. Think of this as a starting point. This is the first step of a journey that will last your entire life. Remember when you were little and your parents would mark your height in some inconspicuous place in the house? Remember how thrilling it was to see how much you had grown from the previous measurement? Remember being a young adult and seeing those markings? We are now going to do something very similar. It is imperative that you make a record of this, your starting point. I encourage you to use this book as a log or journal and have provided space for your notations.

These measurements will only require a tape measure used by tailors or seamstresses and a means to measure your body-fat percentage. The tape measure will be used for several different measurements of various muscle groups. You will measure the biceps, the forearms, the thighs the calves, the hips, the waist, the chest at the top of the ribs just below the clavicle, and the chest with the arms taken at nipple height. These measurements are essential both to mark your progress and also to note areas that may need concentrated effort. You may notice that the right bicep is larger than the left bicep or that your left thigh has a larger circumference than your right thigh. This is all very normal but important to note. The goal is to create symmetry for your body. The right side of your body should be the same size as the left. This is accomplished by working towards your weaker side when you begin your weight training. This means that you should only lift as much with your strong side as the weak side can manage. You will do only as many repetitions of an exercise on the strong side as the weak side can maintain. After only a brief period of time, the weak side will, in a sense, "catch up" to the strong side. From there, you may build on this newly found sense of balance.

Measure your body fat. This measurement determines the portion of your total weight on the scale that is composed of fat. No matter how lean you are (or aren't), you will almost always want to decrease the portion of your total weight that is made up of fat, and increase the portion of your weight that is made up of muscle and bone density. As you will not be able to accurately measure your progress by the weight reflected on the scale, this number provides you with a barometer to measure your progress. The most accurate and cost-effective means to have this measurement taken is with a device called a skin-fold caliper. You can usually have your body-fat measurement taken at a local gym, through a certified nutritionist, or even at through your doctor. The measurement should cost between $15 – $35. If you have difficulty finding a professional to take this measurement, you may call A.C.E. at (800) 825–3636, or www.ideafit.com, for a facility nearest you.

BEFORE

It is extremely important to be clear about where you are at this moment of your transformation. If you allow yourself to take an honest and objective look at yourself at this starting point, you can set and achieve reasonable goals, and you will be best able to assess your progress towards those goals.

Weight on the scale _____

Body-fat percentage _____

Right Bicep _____   Left Bicep _____

Right Forearm _____   Left Forearm _____

Chest (taken at nipple height) _____

Chest with Arms (taken just below the clavicle
   at the top of the rib cage) _____

Waist _____

Hips _____

Right Thigh _____   Left Thigh _____

Right Calf _____   Left Calf _____

If you happen to experience any negative thoughts during your measuring process, take a mental note of those feelings before dismissing them. I ask that you ponder these thoughts briefly so that you can recall precisely the variety of negativism that you will be freeing yourself of. You may notice that these negative thoughts have had severe repercussions in many facets of your life and have negatively affected a healthy self-image. Take note of these negative feelings, as they are about to change. After making your mental notes, let these thoughts go. They are neither an effective motivational tool nor are they useful in building positivity in any way, shape, or form.

It is my understanding that you want to change your body, and by changing your body, ultimately change your life. Making these sweeping changes takes a commitment. I will guide you during this step-by-step process and make it as easy as possible to follow the directions, but it is you who must commit to following these directions to the letter. As you begin Phase One, you need to make a concerted effort to become consistent in your workouts. It is not enough to say that you want to do this. You need to make a promise to yourself and make the commitment of **when** you are going to do it. As you begin this first phase, the goal is to incorporate regular exercise consistently into your schedule. Phase One will last four weeks and requires that you exercise three days per week. I recommend adhering to a Monday/Wednesday/Friday or a Tuesday/Thursday/Saturday schedule. Scheduling your workouts like this helps to accelerate your metabolism and also gives your body the time needed to rest and repair itself. Working out on this type of schedule will also insure that you will not rest for more than two days. If you choose to rest for three days, your metabolism will return to a slower pace and you will not enjoy the maximum potential of the Hot Point program. While on this program, you may choose a longer aerobic workout or to add extra aerobic sessions. Remember that you may do aerobic training up to six days per week, but it is essential that you rest your body, without engaging in any aerobic or weight training, for at least one full day. Pull out your calendar or organizer and commit to scheduling your workouts for the next two weeks—NOW.

Write the dates that you have committed to in the space provided below. Make sure to include the month, day, and year. Filling in the empty spaces below will serve as a binding contract between you and yourself.

Week One   Week Two

_____   _____

_____   _____

_____   _____

The First Two Weeks

The first two weeks of this program will be the most difficult. But if you can stick it out for two weeks, your chances of successfully attaining your goals and completing your physical transformation are exponentially higher. These two weeks are crucial to incorporating this program into your lifestyle. You have made two very significant strides already. You have taken an honest look at where you are at in the process, defining this moment as your starting point, and you have also made a time commitment to bring about the changes that you desire. This mental commitment is vital, but it is your physical willingness that is even more crucial. These first two weeks will test your will, but if you can persevere, you can taste a victory that is sweet indeed.

If you do not exercise regularly, you will experience some soreness during these first two weeks. There is a tremendous difference between the pain associated with injury and the soreness that you will experience the day after a workout. The normal pain associated with exercise and the pain you may encounter during these first two weeks have two distinct sources. Physiologically, when we lift weights, the process of fatiguing the muscle will cause microscopic tearing within the muscle tissue. In the days following a stringent workout, you may experience some stiffness or soreness due to this phenomenon. As these tears heal and repair themselves, the muscle tissue becomes denser and, as a result, will become more defined and can even grow larger in size. During this physiological process of repair, a substance called lactic acid is secreted into the muscle. Lactic acid is a microscopic crystalline substance that has rough, jagged, and pointed edges. When you move, flexing or stretching the muscle in any way, this substance causes a sensation like soreness.

For both of these symptoms, there are several single remedies or combinations that work very effectively to reduce the pain. The first solution would be to take a common pain reliever such as aspirin, Tylenol, ibuprofen, or Naproxen within two hours of your workout. Extra-strength Alka-Seltzer is also very effective at eliminating minor discomforts and helping to combat lactic acid buildup. You should not take these pain relievers regularly for longer than one week. Another very effective method to relieve the soreness associated with exercise is to soak your body in a bathtub of hot water and a healthy dose of Epsom salts. The buildup of lactic acid can also be offset by increasing the amount of water you are drinking. Water is an amazing catalyst to eliminate both lactic acid buildup and to flush fat from the body. As I said, 8–10 glasses is a great start, but working your way up to a gallon a day is even better.

Another obstacle that you may face is fatigue. During these first two weeks you will be asking your body to perform a variety of tasks that it is not used to performing. There is no way to gauge how long this feeling of fatigue may last, but it will certainly not last indefinitely. You may be completely exhausted after your first few sessions, but in time your workouts will have the exact opposite effect. Instead of feeling sluggish after your workout, you will feel completely energized. Take a few choice mental notes as you begin your program if you happen to feel fatigued or sluggish. In four weeks, this will be exactly how you feel if you *don't* work out. Many people I have trained report to feel far less fatigued, sluggish, and sore when they perform aerobic training immediately after weight training. No matter what the obstacle, force yourself to exercise and to complete your session during these first two weeks. By the end of this period, I promise that the pain associated with exercise will have drastically diminished or disappeared altogether, that you will feel energized, and that you will look forward to your next session. The most important thing you can do during these first two weeks is not to quit on yourself.

If you have ever hired a personal trainer, chances are that the trainer has tried to impress you by displaying what a taskmaster he or she is. During their first session with you, most personal trainers will try to push your body very hard. More often than not, you will be so sore the next day that you will think twice before going to your next sessions if you ever go again. Rather than shocking your body to such an extent that you are turned off to exercise, you may want to consider gradually increasing your strength and endurance so that you can achieve the prescribed level of fitness. I am not saying that you shouldn't push yourself or feel that your muscles aren't exhausted at the end of each set . . . I am saying that it is entirely possible that you are not yet capable of maintaining the levels of aerobic or weight training that I am asking you to perform.

Getting Ready for Phase One

If you have never worked out before, there is a possibility that you will not be physically able to do everything that is prescribed. If you are not able to complete either the aerobic or weight training portion of Phase One, don't worry about it, just do what you can. If you cannot perform 20 consecutive minutes of aerobic exercise, make this your goal before you even begin the program. Think of it as your pre–Phase One workout. If you fall into this category, I strongly urge you to purchase and use a heart rate monitor. My experience is that many people perform their aerobics at a rate that is impossible to maintain. They may be on a machine next to someone else and attempt to keep up at a rate of movement that is completely inappropriate for them. If your heart rate gets too elevated, you will not be able to maintain your activity. Learning to keep your heart rate within the target range of 60% – 80% has changed the way many people think and feel about aerobics. Many people who have difficulty adhering to regular aerobic exercise are often elevating their heart rate to anaerobic levels.

When they bring it down into the target range, they not only can perform regular exercise but they actually look forward to it. If you cannot complete the resistance training, again, you will need to gradually increase your strength or stamina until you can complete the prescribed workout. When you attain the level of fitness required to complete the prescribed workout, you will have officially begun Phase One.

Each prescribed exercise will have a corresponding page number on which you will find a description and a photographic example. During these first two weeks, we will utilize aerobic and resistance training to establish a new, and more active, lifestyle. Each workout session will be split up into distinct categories: Aerobic Training, Weight Training, Stretching, and Abdominal Training. Over the next two weeks, your workout will be increased incrementally to insure that you are being challenged and that you are not doing too much as you first begin. After your first two weeks, you can safely incorporate your nutritional program without completely shocking your system.

What you are about to do is really a leap of faith. You have to put a certain level of trust in the fact that this information represents the most cutting edge and scientifically sound information that is available. You have to trust that what I am asking you to do and the direction that I give you will take you from point A to point B. You have to trust that, based on my experience and the results that this program has gotten for thousands, it will also work for you. You also have to trust yourself. You have to be your own taskmaster. You have to push, cajole, and nurture yourself to follow my directions to the letter and push yourself to give 100% of your effort. As your trainer, it is my duty to work myself out of a job. I am training you to be your own personal trainer. Since I am not there to push you into those last few repetitions or to make sure that you complete your aerobics or to watch what you eat, you must be your own coach. I put my faith in you and know that you are the best person for the job.

During these first two weeks you want to make every effort to set yourself up to succeed. You should not try to change too many areas of your life at the same time, so during this first phase we will work towards an end result gradually. The point is to incorporate exercise into your life . . . to look forward to being active. To love being active. To feel the need to be active. To understand that you can push yourself, and when you do, that you can achieve. To experience that you have the power to do something extraordinary.

Day 1

Today is truly the first day of the rest of your life. I encourage you to take a lesson from one of my clients and read through today's exercise prescription, then visualize yourself doing each set of each exercise. Throughout Phase One, I want you to bring this book to the gym with you and check off each set of each exercise as it is completed. Bringing this book should not make you feel self-conscious in any way. In fact, it is not uncommon for many people to have a workout designed for them and have notes available for them to refer to.

The first thing you need to do is to warm up your body. ***Do not stretch before you begin***. You will stretch after each exercise. Instead, choose a machine to do a short, but fairly intense, session of aerobic training.

_____ 5 Minutes of continuous Aerobic Exercise

Let's now begin your first weight training session. On the following page you will see a list of exercises. Each exercise listed will prescribe a certain number of repetitions and a certain number of sets. Next to each exercise is a page number that refers to a detailed description and photographic example of each of the exercises you will encounter. There is also a corresponding stretch for each exercise, which is demonstrated directly after the description of the exercise. You never want to waste time, or rest, once you begin your weight training session. Instead, you will be stretching the muscles that were just exerted. You will also note that there is a blank space for you to fill in, once you determine how heavy your lift will be. To determine the amount of weight you should be lifting, make certain that you can perform the prescribed number of repetitions. If, for instance, the exercise prescribes ten repetitions, make certain that the last three are difficult to move. (Difficult, not impossible.) If the exercise requires twenty reps, the last five should be difficult. In both of these examples, you are using the first 2/3 of the exercise as a warm-up to call upon 100% of your muscle's capability, and reach an anaerobic level in your workout. This is the place where results happen. The last third of each set will determine how dramatic your physical transformation will be. If, during the exercise, your muscles become so exhausted that you simply cannot push the weight, try to concentrate on your breathing and give it your all for one last repetition. If this does not work, lower the weight slightly and finish out the set. Once you have finished the prescribed number of sets for each exercise along with its corresponding stretch, mark ( ) the exercise complete in the space provided.

Note: In the Reps column, M=men, W=women

DAY 1

5 Minute Aerobic Warm-Up ___

Weight Training

Exercise	Demo on pg	Reps	# of Sets	Weight	Stretch on pg	(✓)
Leg Extensions	(41)	M:10 W:20	3 2	_____	(40)	___
Leg Press	(53)	M:10 W:20	3 2	_____	(56)	___
Leg Curls	(43)	M:10 W:20	3 2	_____	(46)	___
Inner Thigh	(47)	20	2	_____		___
Outer Thigh	(48)	20	2	_____		___
Flat Bench Dumbbell Press	(81)	M:10 W:20	3 2	_____	(82)	___
W Shoulders	(94)	M:10 W:20	3 2	_____	(95)	___
Tricep Pushdown	(105)	M:10 W:20	3 2	_____	(102)	___
Curls	(109)	M:10 W:20	3 2	_____	(110)	___

Abdominal Training

Exercise	Demo on pg	Reps	# of Sets	(✓)
Crunches	(60)	20	2	___
Bicycles	(65)	20	2	___
Toe Touches	(63)	20	2	___

20 Minutes of Aerobic Training ___

DAY 2

5 Minute Aerobic Warm-Up   ___

Weight Training

Exercise	Demo on pg	Reps	# of Sets	Weight	Stretch on pg	(✓)
Leg Curls	(43)	M:10	3	_____	(46)	___
		W:20	2			
Leg Extensions	(41)	M:10	3	_____	(40)	___
		W:20	2			
Leg Press	(53)	M:10	3	_____	(56)	___
		W:20	2			
Standing Calf Raise	(50)	20	2	_____	(50)	___
Inclined Bench Press	(83)	M:10	3	_____	(82)	___
		W:20	2			
Lat Pull Down	(71)	M:10	3	_____	(72)	___
		W:20	2			
Lateral Raise	(98)	M:10	3	_____	(95)	___
		W:20	2			
Tricep Extensions	(101)	M:10	3	_____	(102)	___
		W:20	2			
Hammer Curls	(112)	M:10	3	_____	(110)	___
		W:20	2			

Abdominal Training

Exercise	Demo on pg	Reps	# of Sets	(✓)
Diagonal Crunch	(67)	20	2	___
Butt Lifts	(64)	20	2	___
Hand Crunch	(62)	20	2	___

20 Minutes of Aerobic Training   ___

DAY 3

5 Minute Aerobic Warm-Up   ___

Weight Training

Exercise	Demo on pg	Reps	# of Sets	Weight	Stretch on pg	(✓)
Leg Press	(53)	M:10 W:20	2 3	_____	(56)	___
Leg Curls	(43)	M:10 W:20	2 3	_____	(46)	___
Outer Thigh	(48)	20	2	_____	(49)	___
Inner Thigh	(47)	20	2	_____	(48)	___
Seated Calf Raise	(51)	20	2	_____	(51)	___
W Shoulders	(94)	M:10 W:20	3 2	_____	(95)	___
Seated Row	(73)	M:10 W:20	3 2	_____	(72)	___
Overhead Tricep Extension	(103)	M:10 W:20	3 2	_____	(102)	___
Concentration Curls	(111)	M:10 W:20	3 2	_____	(110)	___

Abdominal Training

Exercise	Demo on pg	Reps	# of Sets	(✓)
Penguins	(66)	20	2	___
Side Crunches	(68)	20	2	___
Toe Touches	(63)	20	2	___

20 Minutes of Aerobic Training   ___

5 Minute Aerobic Warm-Up   ___

Weight Training

Exercise	Demo on pg	Reps	# of Sets	Weight	Stretch on pg	(✓)
Push-ups	(87)	M:20 W:20	3 2	_____	(82)	___
Tricep Kickbacks with a Twist	(106)	M:10 W:20	3 2	_____	(102)	___
One Arm Row	(75)	M:10 W:20	3 2	_____	(72)	___
Goal Posts	(96)	20	3	_____	(95)	___
Inner Thigh	(47)	20	2	_____		___
Outer Thigh	(48)	20	2	_____		___
Squat #1	(55)	M:10 W:20	3 2	_____	(56)	___
Walking Lunges	(39)	20 paces	2	_____	(40)	___
Leg Curls	(43)	M:10 W:20	3 2	_____	(40)	___

Abdominal Training

Exercise	Demo on pg	Reps	# of Sets	(✓)
Crunches	(60)	20	2	___
Diagonal Crunch	(67)	20	2	___
Bicycles	(65)	20	2	___

20 Minutes of Aerobic Training   ___

DAY 5

5 Minute Aerobic Warm-Up   ___

Weight Training

Exercise	Demo on pg	Reps	# of Sets	Weight	Stretch on pg	(✓)
Seated Calf Raise	(51)	20	2	_____		___
Leg Extensions	(41)	M:10	3	_____	(40)	___
		W:20	2			
Leg Curls	(43)	M:10	3	_____	(46)	___
		W:20	2			
Walking Lunges	(34)	20 paces	2		(40)	___
Triceps Push-down	(105)	M:10	3	_____	(102)	___
		W:20	2			
Lat Pull Down	(71)	M:10	2	_____	(72)	___
		W:20	2			
Delt Wing	(97)	M:10	3	_____	(95)	___
		W:20	2			
Cable Curls	(113)	M:10	3	_____	(110)	___
		W:20	2			

Abdominal Training

Exercise	Demo on pg	Reps	# of Sets	(✓)
Penguins	(66)	20	2	___
Hand Crunches	(62)	20	2	___
Butt Lift	(64)	20	2	___

20 Minutes of Aerobic Training   ___

DAY 6

5 Minute Aerobic Warm-Up _____

Weight Training

Exercise	Demo on pg	Reps	# of Sets	Weight	Stretch on pg	(✓)
C sweep	(91)	M:10	3	_____	(82)	___
		W:20	2			
Tricep Extension	(101)	M:10	3	_____	(102)	___
		W:20	2			
Seated Row	(73)	M:10	3	_____	(72)	___
		W:20	2			
Lateral Raise	(98)	M:10	3	_____	(95)	___
		W:20	2			
Curls	(109)	M:10	3	_____	(110)	___
		W:20	2			
Butt Kicks	(52)	20	2	_____	(46)	___
Leg Curls	(43)	M:10	3	_____	(46)	___
		W:20	2			
Leg Press	(53)	M:10	3	_____	(56)	___
		W:20	2			
Standing Calf Raise	(50)	20	2	_____		___

Abdominal Training

Exercise	Demo on pg	Reps	# of Sets	(✓)
Roman Sit-Ups	(61)	20	2	___
Side Crunch	(68)	20	2	___
Bicycles	(65)	20	2	___

20 Minutes of Aerobic Training _____

HALFWAY POINT

The most difficult part of your transformation is over. I want you to take a moment and give yourself a well-deserved pat on the back. You have successfully completed the first half of the first phase, and you are on the road to seeing some significant results. At this point you should definitely feel the difference in your muscles, and may even be seeing some changes in the mirror. This is exciting stuff, so take this time to note your accomplishments to date.

The second half of the first phase is only slightly different than the two weeks you have just completed. Up until now, your program consisted of aerobic training, resistance training, stretching, and abdominal training. During the next two weeks, you will attempt to add five more minutes to your aerobic training (now you will be performing 25 minutes of aerobic training). If you can, continue to work out on a Monday/Wednesday/Friday or a Tuesday/Thursday/Saturday schedule. It is now time to add the last third of the puzzle. Up until this point, it was imperative not to completely shock your system, and to familiarize your body with the demands of exercise. Now you are ready for the rest. The final third of this program to incorporate into your daily life is a nutritional program that you can live with, that makes sense, and that is easy to adhere to.

The goal of this process is to let your old facade melt into the body you desire. Regardless of whether you want to tone your muscles or increase your size, it is imperative that you reduce your body-fat percentage, and it is vital to eliminate the amount of fat underneath your skin. To accomplish this, you will now need to incorporate the nutritional portion of this program into your daily regimen.

As you begin your nutritional program, I again ask that you jump into it without testing the water. I plead with you to re-read Chapter Five and gain a complete understanding of your new nutritional program. It can be as easy or complex as you like. Again, you are creating a positive habit, and forming that habit takes a little time. If you start your eating program today, in two weeks when you complete Phase One, your new diet will become second nature to you. In two weeks you will have a keen understanding of what your body needs for food and when you will need to eat. You will find that your energy level will be even, without the highs and lows you may now experience during the course of your day. You will have a real and tangible feeling when and how fast you are burning calories off and just how much you have accelerated your metabolism. Putting together a comprehensive program that includes aerobic training, resistance training, and a sound nutritional program will indeed change the way you look. Incorporating these three components into your life will alter the way you physically feel and will completely transform the way you feel about yourself.

At this point in your training, and from this point on, you may be seeing some puzzling changes in your body. There is just no way to be certain where you are going to see this change first. While some may first notice weight loss in the face, others experience reductions just above their "love handles," and others still may notice their loss in their upper chest. Often when we first notice weight loss, we are alarmed because the reduction accentuates a portion of the body just above or below, making us *look* fatter. Your eyes are just playing tricks on you. The fact of the matter is that there is no way to predict where we are going to lose those first few pounds of fat. It is important to realize that indeed you have lost some fat, and to have the confidence that you will lose much more. This is not lyposuction, and spot reduction is a myth. In time you will reduce your body-fat percentage dramatically, and this overall reduction will begin to spread out more evenly as more time passes.

Before you begin your next two weeks of the program, consult your calendar or organizer, and commit to your next six sessions

Make a notation of the month, day and year, along with the time you are committing to be at the gym.

Do not let anything come between you and this commitment.

Day 7 _____ at _____   Day 10 _____ at _____

Day 8 _____ at _____   Day 11 _____ at _____

Day 9 _____ at _____   Day 12 _____ at _____

DAY 7

5 Minute Aerobic Warm-Up ___

Weight Training

Exercise	Demo on pg	Reps	# of Sets	Weight	Stretch on pg	(✓)
Leg Extensions	(41)	M:10	3	_____	(40)	___
		W:20	2			
Squat #1	(55)	20	2	_____	(56)	___
Leg Curls	(45)	M:10	3	_____	(46)	___
		W:20	2			
Inner Thigh	(47)	20	2	_____		___
Outer Thigh	(48)	20	2	_____		___
Push-ups	(87)	M:10	2	_____	(82)	___
		W:20	2			
One Arm Row	(75)	M:10	3	_____	(72)	___
		W:20	2			
Front Raise	(99)	M:10	3	_____	(95)	___
		W:20	2			
Tricep Extension	(101)	M:10	3	_____	(102)	___
		W:20	2			
Hammer Curls	(112)	M:10	3	_____	(110)	___
		W:20	2			

Abdominal Training

Exercise	Demo on pg	Reps	# of Sets	(✓)
Crunches	(60)	20	3	___
Side Crunch	(68)	20	3	___
Toe Touches	(63)	20	3	___

25 Minutes of Aerobic Training ___

DAY 8

5 Minute Aerobic Warm-Up   —

Weight Training

Exercise	Demo on pg	Reps	# of Sets	Weight	Stretch on pg	(✓)
Flat Bench Press	(81)	M:10 W:20	3 2	_____	(82)	—
Overhead Tricep Extension	(103)	W:20 M:10	3 3	_____	(102)	—
W Shoulders	(94)	W:20 M:10	3 3	_____	(95)	—
Hyper-extension	(77)	W:10 M:10	3 3	_____	(72)	—
Concentration Curls	(111)	M:10 W:20	3 2	_____	(110)	—
Leg Curls	(43)	W:20 M:10	2 2	_____	(46)	—
Squat #1	(55)	W:20 M:10	2 2	_____	(56)	—
Walking Lunges	(39)	20 Paces	2		(40)	—
Standing Calf Raise	(50)	20	2	_____		—
Butt Kicks	(52)	20	2	_____	(46)	—

Abdominal Training

Exercise	Demo on pg	Reps	# of Sets	(✓)
Butt Lifts	(64)	20	3	—
Penguins	(66)	20	3	—
Hand Crunches	(62)	20	3	—
Roman Chair	(61)	20	3	—

25 Minutes of Aerobic Training   —

DAY 9

5 Minute Aerobic Warm-Up _____

Weight Training

Exercise	Demo on pg	Reps	# of Sets	Weight	Stretch on pg	(✓)
Squat #2	(57)	M:10 W:20	3 2	_____	(56)	___
Leg Curls	(43)	M:10 W:20	3 2	_____	(46)	___
Leg Extensions	(41)	M:10 W:20	3 2	_____	(40)	___
Walking Lunges	(39)	20 Paces	2		(40)	___
Seated Calf Raise	(51)	20	2	_____		___
Lat Pull Down	(71)	M:10 W:20	3 2	_____	(72)	___
Goal Post	(96)	20	3	_____	(95)	___
Incline Fly	(85/86)	M:10 W:20	3 2	_____	(82)	___
Bench Dips	(104)	M:10 W:20	3 2	_____	(102)	___
Cable Curls	(113)	M:10 W:20	3 2	_____	(110)	___

Abdominal Training

Exercise	Demo on pg	Reps	# of Sets	(✓)
Bicycles	(65)	20	3	___
Diagonal Crunch	(67)	20	3	___
Side Crunch	(68)	20	3	___

25 Minutes of Aerobic Training _____

DAY 10

5 Minute Aerobic Warm-Up   ___

Weight Training

Exercise	Demo on pg	Reps	# of Sets	Weight	Stretch on pg	(✔)
Pec Deck	(84)	M:10 W:20	3 2	_____	(82)	___
Tricep Kickback with Twist	(106)	M:10 W:20	3 2	_____	(102)	___
Seated Row	(73)	M:10 W:20	3 2	_____	(72)	___
Lateral Raise	(98)	M:10 W:20	3 2	_____	(95)	___
Inner Thigh	(47)	20	2	_____		___
Outer Thigh	(48)	20	2	_____		___
Butt Kicks	(52)	20	2	_____	(56)	___
Leg Extensions	(41)	M:10 W:20	3 2	_____	(40)	___
Leg Press	(53)	M:10 W:20	3 2	_____	(56)	___
Standing Calf Raise	(50)	20	2	_____	(50)	___

Abdominal Training

Exercise	Demo on pg	Reps	# of Sets	(✔)
Roman Sit-ups	(61)	20	3	___
Toe Touches	(63)	20	3	___
Butt Lift	(64)	20	3	___

25 Minutes of Aerobic Training   ___

DAY 11

5 Minute Aerobic Warm-Up _____

Weight Training

Exercise	Demo on pg	Reps	# of Sets	Weight	Stretch on pg	(✓)
Squat #2	(57)	M:10 W:20	3 2	_____	(56)	___
Leg Curls	(43)	M:10 W:20	3 2	_____	(46)	___
Outer Thigh	(48)	20	3	_____	(48)	___
Inner Thigh	(47)	20	3	_____	(47)	___
Walking Lunge	(39)	20 Paces	2	_____	(40)	___
Push-ups	(87)	M:10 W:20	3 2	_____	(82)	___
One Arm Row	(75)	M:10 W:20	3 2	_____	(72)	___
Delt Wing	(97)	M:10 W:20	3 2	_____	(95)	___
Tricep Kickback with a Twist	(106)	M:10 W:20	3 2	_____	(110)	___
Curls	(109)	M:10 W:20	3 2	_____	(110)	___

Abdominal Training

Exercise	Demo on pg	Reps	# of Sets	(✓)
Bicycles	(65)	20	3	___
Penguins	(66)	20	3	___
Hand Crunch	(62)	20	3	___

25 Minutes of Aerobic Training _____

5 Minute Aerobic Warm-Up   ___

Weight Training

Exercise	Demo on Pg	Reps	# of Sets	Weight	Stretch on pg	(✓)
Tricep Push-downs	(105)	M:10	3	_____	(110)	___
		W:20	2			
C Sweep	(91)	M:10	3	_____	(82)	___
		W:20	2			
Front Raise	(99)	M:10	3	_____	(95)	___
		W:20	2			
Shrugs	(79)	M:20	3	_____	(72)	___
		W:20	2			
Hammer Curls	(112)	M:10	3	_____	(110)	___
		W:20	2			
Leg Extensions	(41)	M:10	3	_____	(40)	___
		W:20	2			
Butt Kicks	(52)	20	2	_____	(46)	___
Leg Press	(53)	M:10	3	_____	(56)	___
		W:20	2			
Walking Lunges	(39)	20 Paces	2	_____	(40)	___
Standing Calf Raise	(50)	20	2	_____	(50)	___

Abdominal Training

Exercise	Demo on pg	Reps	# of Sets	(✓)
Diagonal Crunches	(67)	20	3	___
Side Crunch	(68)	20	3	___
Toe Touches	(63)	20	3	___

25 Minutes of Aerobic Training   ___

FINISH LINE

Congratulations! You have completed Phase One. This is a time for celebration.

This celebration should also involve some honest reflection. How do you feel today, as opposed to just four short weeks ago? Remember when you took your measurements and considered any negative thoughts that were present in your head? Are you free of those negative thoughts? How do you think you look? How do your clothes fit? What is your energy level like now, as opposed to when you first started the program? Compare your job or scholastic performance to that of four weeks ago. Do words like "desire" and "drive" have a different meaning for you today, as opposed to when you first started? How does it feel for you to set and meet a certain set of goals several times a week? Has your image of yourself or the respect you have for yourself changed over the last four weeks?

Take a really close look at these numbers. Can you now see what a little effort can result in? When you began this program, you had a vision of what you would like your body to look like and you set some goals. If you have not achieved your ultimate goals, how close did you get? How much progress have you made?

The most important thing you have accomplished is that you have incorporated exercise and a new way of eating into your life. Because you have exercised regularly for four weeks, this routine should now be a habit. Habits are addicting, so be forewarned that soon you are going to be craving your workouts, and that urge will only become stronger. Unlike any other addiction, this one is good for you. This addiction creates euphoria, improves your sexual drive, makes you feel fantastic, helps you sleep, and will leave you looking better and better each time you get your fix. What is even more intoxicating, however, is that in just one short hour you will have set and attained many goals. The intoxication of achievement and success, and the momentum this creates, will reverberate throughout your life and positively affect every aspect of it. What you are now experiencing is truly a positive addiction.

What Next?

At this point, it is important to determine what you would like to do next, and determine what level of fitness you would like to attain. You may want to take your workouts to a higher level and feel that it is time for a new challenge. You may find that your personal time constraints or the goals you have set for yourself can be accommodated by the three-days-per-week workout schedule of Phase One.

Some of you may be very comfortable working out three days per week, and find that your goals and needs are met by the Phase One level of exercise. For some, attaining this level of fitness has been a minor miracle, and has given you a quality of life you have been yearning for. Others still, especially the elderly, find that this schedule enables you to have confidence in yourself and your movement, has allowed you to regain muscle strength, reverses osteoporosis, and makes you feel revitalized and energetic.

If you desire a new challenge and want to take your physical transformation to the next level, Phase Two will suit you. If you choose to advance to Phase Two, you will be exercising four days per week, and each session will last approximately fifteen minutes longer than your present sessions.

If you choose to remain in Phase One, there are several adjustments you will need to make, insuring that you will continue to experience results and avoid reaching a training plateau. By this time you will have realized that no two workouts you have performed to this point have been the same. The reason your workouts have been structured in this way was to continually surprise your body, and to prevent you from working out in the same manner on successive days. You may repeat the workouts in Phase One over and over again. I strongly suggest that every two weeks you increase your aerobic workout by five minutes. And do more than one hour and fifteen minutes. After your third cycle, invert the order of excercises prescribed each day. After three cycles, you may shuffle the cycles slightly. Look to the "Hot Point Resistance Training" section in Chapter Four, and introduce a new excercise into your routine each week. Then repeat the entire process. By merely switching the order of weight training exercises, you will continually shock the muscles and never become bored in your workouts.

It is now time for you to see your progress on paper.

AFTER

It is so important to be clear about where you are at this moment of your transformation and to be keenly aware of just how far you have come. Allowing yourself to see what you have accomplished in only four weeks will enable you set new goals for what you would like to accomplish next.

Weight on the scale _____
Body fat percentage _____
Right Bicep _____   Left Bicep _____
Right Forearm _____   Left Forearm _____
Chest (taken at nipple height) _____
Chest with Arms (taken just below the clavicle
   at the top of the rib cage) _____
Waist _____
Hips _____
Right Thigh _____   Left Thigh _____
Right Calf _____   Left Calf _____

Take a moment to compare the numbers you have just written with the numbers you inserted on the "Before" page four weeks ago.

8

Phase Two—4 day a week workout routines

If you have just completed Phase One, you may skip ahead to page 184 and begin this chapter just after the measurements. If you are using Phase Two as your starting point, I will assume that you are already pretty fit and are exercising several times a week and already training with weights four times per week. What you are about to embark upon is completely different than what you are currently doing.

Hot Point Fitness is a three-pronged attack designed to completely transform your body. Since you are already exercising and have purchased this book, let's examine the reasons for your purchase. Maybe you are an exercise junkie or a professional trainer, and you just want to read another opinion on what may be the best strategy for exercise. If this is the case, I would suggest that merely reading my strategy does not truly provide the information that you need. You need to experience these workouts for yourself to gauge just how revolutionary this program is. For those readers who may actually be trainers, I strongly suggest that, as an experiment, you put yourself in the shoes of a trainee and follow the directions exactly like you would expect one of your clients to follow yours. Carefully read the directions before each resistance exercise, then perform it to the letter. I promise that even you will experience a physical transformation. If you are, on the other hand, a person who is currently working out four times per week, chances are that you purchased this book because you have come to a crossroads of sorts and are no longer experiencing the results you desire. You are spending much of your time, and you are putting in so much effort to achieve a goal, and yet, for one reason or another, you are not getting the results you desire. If you fall into this category, have no fear, your results are on the way.

Most people who exercise and exercise regularly are not seeing results. The next time you are at the gym, take a look around. The person on the Stair Master next to you might have been coming into the gym for many years, but do they look any different than when you first saw them? Probably not. The person who you see weight training, who is there almost religiously, is not enjoying any significant results either. When you look in the mirror, you may share their frustration. The problem lies not in your commitment, but rather in the method that you have been employing to achieve the results you desire.

After your first set you will discover how truly different this program is. You may have to drop the weight that you would normally lift so significantly that you might become discouraged. Almost every professional athlete that I have ever trained is tremendously shocked when they first begin to work with me. Their chief complaint is, "I used to be able to lift twice what I am lifting now with no problem at all. I am getting weaker instead of stronger. This just isn't working." The reason they were able to move so much more weight before is that they were using momentum, or swinging the weights, and not doing the exercises properly. They called upon several other muscles or muscle groups to help them move the weight. In essence, they were not really working the muscle that the exercise was intended to work, but were only concentrating on how much weight they could lift, as if that were the goal. They were defeating themselves by trying to lift so much. They really were not working the intended muscle in any of their exercises. Remember, it is not how much weight you move, but rather how impeccable the technique. If you find yourself getting frustrated because you are used to moving a great deal more weight, be patient. Your weight will go back up to where it was, and then even higher. Not only will you become much stronger by implementing Hot Point, but your strength will be more evenly distributed.

Another reason those who exercise regularly do not experience more dramatic results is that they perform almost the exact same exercises in the exact same order each and every time they work out. If you tend to fit into this category, there are a number of things you can do to jump-start your results. Primarily, your chief concern will be to constantly surprise the body by never performing the same workout on two consecutive days. Simply follow the prescribed workouts for the next four weeks. After these four weeks you may simply repeat the workouts. Not only will you find that constantly surprising the body will pay dividends in terms of the way you look, but you will also find that you are more excited by the prospect of working out than you have been for quite some time. Your workout should be as invigorating for your mind as it is for your body. As you are already at a fairly high level of fitness, challenging yourself mentally might just be the missing piece of your puzzle.

Hot Point Fitness is as much about transforming the way you mentally approach your workout and improving your self-image and esteem as it is about transforming your appearance. If you are already training with weights four days per week, you are obviously motivated. If you have not experienced results for quite a while, I have no idea what has motivated you to continue to work out. I can only assume that you have enormous will. For most who start from square one, creating a sense of willpower, achievement, and self-esteem are as rewarding as the amazing physical changes they see in the mirror. For you, it is precisely the continuation of your physical transformation that is and should be your goal. To facilitate this achievement, you must focus a great deal on visualizing that goal. Spend a significant amount of time seeing in your mind's eye exactly what you would look like after you have achieved your goal. I have clients who write their goals down with a deadline date (including month, day, and year), and they post it in a place where they will see it several times per day. I have other clients who create a collage with pictures. Again, they post this in a place where they are forced to see it, and this seems to work. While it may sound strange to some, stating a goal and being reminded of it daily is sometimes very helpful in achieving the stated objective. I have several successful clients who, when they started their businesses, wrote out a check for the amount of money they wanted to make from their venture. Without exception, all of them made nearly the exact dollar figure that they had visualized. Had they known that visualizing their success would be so effective, I think that they would have added an extra zero! Visualization of your intended goal and being constantly reminded of that goal just may be the ammunition that you need to keep going and keep seeing results. It just might give you that singularity of purpose that you need to get over the hump.

The point of this program is to transform your body. Mark today as a starting point. To define this moment, determine your body-fat percentage, and take some measurements of different body parts to understand where you are at right at this moment and also to be able to compare your progress.

If you began with Phase One, you have been exercising for at least four weeks and you have successfully incorporated exercise and nutrition into your lifestyle. Phase Two is the point at which you take your level of physical fitness and physical transformation to a higher level. That lifestyle change should begin to pay some significant dividends. You should have noticed some significant stress relief. You should be experiencing an enhanced self-esteem and a more positive outlook on life. You should be noticing yourself smiling more oftens and you should be feeling very, very good about yourself and what you are doing. You should be noticing some significant changes in your appearance, and you should be feeling that your musculature is becoming better formed, more defined, and perhaps a little larger. If you started with Phase One, I hope that you are looking forward to exercising and coming to find that you have created a new habit that you just cannot live without. You feel great, admit it. You have created a program of regular exercise for yourself and are seeing and feeling a difference. You have completed at least two weeks on your new nutritional program, and those around you are beginning to notice that you look and act differently. You may feel like a completely different person than you did just four short weeks ago. This new habit gives you positive reinforcement, helps you realize that you are a success, enables you to achieve goals on a daily basis, and allows you to feel like a winner. The positive addiction you have created for yourself is spilling over into every aspect of your life. This is great news for you and those around you. Even greater is the news that it just gets better over the next four weeks.

Phase One ends by rechecking your body-fat percentage and retaking measurements. It is important that you understand where you are at right now. Compare where you are at right now with where you were when you started. What are you going to do to reward yourself for your progress? Be sure to reward yourself with something wonderful. You are doing something very special, and this is a special occasion. After rewarding yourself, again look at where you are right now and compare it with where you are going and where you want to go. Is this goal achievable? Would you like to restate your objective? Become very clear and specific with yourself. Spend some time contemplating what it is you want to achieve, and write your goal down. Post this goal in a place where you will see it everyday. I recommend placing your goal on the bathroom mirror or the refrigerator. Better yet, place your goal on both. This way, every time you look in the mirror and see what is happening to your body, you can mentally push yourself to go even further. Every time you go to open the fridge, you can ask yourself if the food you are about to put into your mouth will take you toward your goal or prevent you from achieving it. It is the mental strength that you bring to Phase Two that will ultimately make a difference.

Phase Two requires a new level of commitment to transform your body. It is truly important that your goals be clear and that you utilize your mental toolbox to elevate your level of performance. Calling upon all the tools you have at your disposal will make the process infinitely easier and enhance your results even further. This next phase does not require you to double the amount of time you spend on your workout, but only to double your commitment to the process of transformation. The time spent is increased only fractionally, and yet you may indeed double your results.

Phase Two's level of training is fairly intense. In fact, by exercising at this level, you will quickly be amongst the top 10 percent of Americans in terms of physical fitness. This level of training will help you to attain the physique you desire and allow you to maintain this level of conditioning. When celebrities are not getting ready for a film, and when athletes are not competing for a place on the Olympic team, this is the level at which they would normally train. When they do get that part, or when they need to begin training for an event, they can quickly change gears and take their level of performance to a new level quite easily. Exercising at this level also promotes optimum levels for your cardiovascular, circulatory, and immune systems, bolstering your long-term health. Working out at this level is a recipe for a full, active, and long life.

Phase Two will necessitate scheduling four days for your workout rather than three. During the four days you spend working out, you will increase the amount of aerobic exercise by ten minutes and increase the amount of time you spend weight training by ten minutes. This means that you will be spending a full hour exercising four times per week. You may also decide that you would like to slightly alter your nutritional program to help you achieve new objectives. Nutritional changes should not be radical in any way, but only increase or reduce your total caloric intake by a maximum of 15%. These changes are minor in terms of scheduling and convenience, but will yield major results.

Changing the Workout

Because of the additional demands on your time, you may choose to split your workout up over the day. This is perfectly acceptable, provided that you get your entire workout in. You have the option of splitting up your workout and having considerably less structure than you did in Phase One. You may choose to do your abdominal work in the morning, you may choose to do your aerobics after dinner, you may choose to perform your weight training after work. The choice is yours. Just be sure to find room to complete the entire workout. If you find that on two consecutive workout days you have not completed everything that was prescribed, I urge you to rethink your schedule and attempt to get it all in at the same time. My suggestion is to do them all at once. It is my opinion that the abdominal workout is part of the resistance training, and completing your aerobic activity immediately afterwards will help you to reenergize and flush lactic acid buildup. To find a block of time that accommodates all of this is sometimes not feasible. But if you really look, you have the time. You may work nine hours, you may sleep eight hours, you may spend an hour doing chores around the house, you may spend two hours having quality time with friends and family, you may spend two hours watching television . . . but that still leaves two hours to get your workout in. The point is to fit it into your schedule.

Scheduling

It is time to make a commitment to yourself. Working out at this level will require that you schedule in four days a week for the next four weeks. I suggest that these four sessions be spaced out throughout the week, so that you are never taking off more than two consecutive days. Make a promise to yourself that you will get to the gym eight times during the next two weeks. Consult with your organizer, day planner, or computerized scheduling device and block out your time. Fill in the spaces provided below with dates and times. This will be a binding contract between you and yourself.

DAY 1 _____   DAY 2 _____
DAY 3 _____   DAY 4 _____
DAY 5 _____   DAY 6 _____
DAY 7 _____   DAY 8 _____

With the above schedule written in this book and in your weekly calendar, you are now ready to begin Phase Two of your transformation.

Depending on your goals, you may decide that you need to increase the amount of aerobic activity you are doing and/or the number of days you do that aerobic activity. You may do aerobic and abdominal training for up to six days per week. Again, you need one full day of rest to allow the body to heal. This does not mean that you cannot play a game of golf or take a walk along the beach at sunset or play softball. Simply let your body have a little break so that it can be ready to perform at the highest level possible.

After your first week or two in Phase Two, you might find that you are completely exhausted, or that you aren't motivated enough to make it into the gym. If this happens, it is quite possible that you are overtraining. If your body is overtrained, it does not mean that you have failed in any way. It simply means that your body is not ready at this very moment to make the jump to your next phase. You may choose to push yourself and complete another week at this level. Or you may choose to simply repeat the second half of Phase One. After you repeat the second half of Phase One, try the four-days-per-week workout schedule again, beginning with Day 1.

Note: In the Reps column, M=men, W=women

DAY 1

5 Minute Aerobic Warm-Up ___

Weight Training

Exercise	Demo on pg	Reps	# of Sets	Weight	Stretch on pg	(✓)
Flat Fly	(85)	W:20 M:10	2 3	_____	(82)	___
Incline Press	(83)	W:20 M:10	2 3	_____	(82)	___
Push-ups	(87)	W:20 M:10	2 3	_____	(82)	___
W Shoulders	(94)	W:20 M:10	2 3	_____	(95)	___
Lat Raise	(98)	W:20 M:10	2 3	_____	(95)	___
Delt Wing	(97)	W:20 M:10	2 3	_____	(95)	___
Overhead Tricep Extension	(103)	W:20 M:10	2 3	_____	(102)	___
Bench Dips	(104)	W:20 M:10	3 2	_____	(102)	___
Tricep Push-downs	(105)	W:20 M:10	2 3	_____	(102)	___

Abdominal Training

Exercise	Demo on pg	Reps	# of Sets	(✓)
Crunch	(60)	20	2	___
Bicycles	(65)	20	2	___
Peguins	(66)	20	2	___
Toe Touches	(63)	20	2	___

35 Minutes of Aerobic Training ___

5 Minute Aerobic Warm-Up   ___

Weight Training

Exercise	Demo on pg	Reps	# of Sets	Weight	Stretch on pg	(✓)
Leg Extension	(41)	W:20	2	_____	(40)	___
		M:10	3			
Squat #2	(57)	W:20	2	_____	(56)	___
		M:10	3			
Walking Lunges	(39)	30 paces	2		(40)	___
Lying Leg Curls	(45)	W:20	3	_____	(46)	___
		M:10	3			
Butt Kicks	(52)	20 each leg	3	1 – 5 Pound Ankle Weights		___
Inner Thigh	(47)	20	3		(47)	___
Lat Pull Down	(71)	W:20	2	_____	(72)	___
		M:10	3			
Hyper-extension	(77)	20	3		(72)	___
Curl	(109)	W:20	2	_____	(110)	___
		M:10	3			

Abdominal Training

Exercise	Demo on pg	Reps	# of Sets	(✓)
Hand Crunch	(62)	20	2–3	___
Side Crunch	(68)	20	2–3	___
Roman Chair	(61)	20	2–3	___
Butt Lift	(64)	20	2–3	___

35 Minutes of Aerobic Training   ___

5 Minute Aerobic Warm-Up _____

Weight Training

Exercise	Demo on pg	Reps	# of Sets	Weight	Stretch on pg	(✔)
Pec Deck	(89)	W:20 M:10	2 3	_____	(82)	___
Dumbbell Press (bar optional)	(81)	W:20 M:10	2 3	_____	(82)	___
Decline Fly	(85/86)	W:20 M:10	2 3	_____	(82)	___
W Shoulders	(94)	W:20 M:10	2 3	_____	(95)	___
Front Raise	(99)	W:20 M:10	2 3	_____	(95	___
Goal Posts	(96)	W:20 M:10	2 3	_____	(95)	___
Tricep Kickback with Twist	(106)	W:20 M:10	2 3	_____	(102)	___
Tricep Extension	(101	W:20 M:10	2 3	_____	(102)	___
Tricep Push-downs	(105)	W:20 M:10	2 3	_____	(102)	___

Abdominal Training

Exercise	Demo on pg	Reps	# of Sets	(✔)
Crunch	(60)	20	2–3	___
Bicycles	(65)	20	2–3	___
Penguins	(66)	20	2–3	___
Diagonal Crunch	(67)	20	2–3	___

35 Minutes of Aerobic Training _____

(continues)

DAY 4

5 Minute Aerobic Warm-Up   ___

Weight Training

Exercise	Demo on pg	Reps	# of Sets	Weight	Stretch on pg	(✓)
Leg Curls	(43)	W:20 M:10	2 3	_____	(46)	___
Walking Lunges	(39)	30 Paces	2	_____	(40)	___
Squat #2	(57)	W:20 M:10	2 3	_____	(56)	___
Leg Extension	(41)	W:20 M:10	3 2	_____	(40)	___
Standing Calf Raise	(50)	20	3		(40)	
Seated Row	(73)	W:20 M:10	2 3	_____	(72)	___
One-Arm Row	(75)	W:20 M:10	2 3	_____	(72)	___
Hyperextension	(77)	W:20 M:15	2 3	_____	(72)	___
Cable Curls	(113)	W:20 M:10	2 3	_____	(110)	___
Hammer Curls	(112)	W:20 M:10	2 3	_____	(110)	___

Abdominal Training

Exercise	Demo on pg	Reps	# of Sets	(✓)
Butt Lifts	(64)	20	2–3	___
Side Crunch	(68)	20	2–3	___
Toe Touches	(63)	20	2–3	___
Roman Chair	(61)	20	2–3	___

35 Minutes of Aerobic Training   ___

DAY 5

5 Minute Aerobic Warm-Up _____

Weight Training

Exercise	Demo on pg	Reps	# of Sets	Weight	Stretch on pg	(✓)
Incline Fly	(85/86)	W:20 M:10	2 3	_____	(82)	___
C Sweep	(91)	W:20 M:10	2 3	_____	(82)	___
Push-ups	(87)	W:10 M:20	3 3		(82)	___
Delt Wing	(97)	W:20 M:10	2 3	_____	(95)	___
Lat Raise	(98)	W:20 M:10	2 3	_____	(95)	___
Front Raise	(99)	W:20 M:10	2 3	_____	(95)	___
Bench Dips	(104)	W:10 M:20	2 3		(102)	___
Tricep Pushdowns	(105)	W:20 M:10	2 3	_____	(102)	___
Tricep Kickbacks With a Twist	(106)	W:20 M:10	2 3	_____	(102)	___

Abdominal Training

Exercise	Demo on pg	Reps	# of Sets	(✓)
Hyper-extensions	(77)	20	2–3	___
Bicycles	(65)	20	2–3	___
Penguins	(66)	20	2–3	___
Hand Crunch	(62)	20	2–3	___

35 Minutes of Aerobic Training _____

DAY 6

5 Minute Aerobic Warm-Up   ___

Weight Training

Exercise	Demo on pg	Reps	# of Sets	Weight	Stretch on pg	(✓)
Walking Lunges	(39)	20 Paces	3		(40)	___
Leg Curls	(45)	W:20 M:10	2 3	_____	(46)	___
Leg Press	(53)	W:20 M:10	2 3	_____	(56)	___
Inner Thigh	(47)	20	2	_____	(47)	___
Outer Thigh	(48)	20	2	_____	(48)	___
One Arm Row	(75)	W:20 M:10	2 3	_____	(72)	___
Lat Pull Down	(71)	W:20 M:10	2 3	_____	(72)	___
Shrugs	(79)	20	3	_____	(72)	___
Concentric Curl	(111)	W:20 M:10	2 3	_____	(110)	___
Curls	(109)	W:20 M:10	2 3	_____	(110)	___

Abdominal Training

Exercise	Demo on pg	Reps	# of Sets	(✓)
Roman Sit-ups	(61)	20	2–3	___
Toe Touches	(63)	20	2–3	___
Side Crunch	(68)	20	2–3	___
Butt Lift	(64)	20	2–3	___

35 Minutes of Aerobic Training   ___

DAY 7

5 Minute Aerobic Warm-Up   ___

Weight Training

Exercise	Demo on pg	Reps	# of Sets	Weight	Stretch on pg	(✓)
Pec Deck	(89)	W:20	2	_____	(82)	___
		M:10	3			
Decline Press	(84)	W:20	2	_____	(82)	___
		M:10	3			
Incline Press	(83)	W:20	2	_____	(82)	___
		M:10	3			
Goal Posts	(96)	W:20	2	_____	(95)	___
		M:10	3			
W Shoulders	(94)	W:20	2	_____	(95)	___
		M:10	3			
Lat Raise	(98)	W:20	2	_____	(95)	___
		M:10	3			
Tricep Push-down	(105)	W:20	2	_____	(102)	___
		M:10	3			
Bench Dips	(104)	20	3	_____	(102)	___
Overhead Tricep	(103)	W:20	2	_____	(102)	___
Extension		M:10	3			

Abdominal Training

Exercise	Demo on pg	Reps	# of Sets	(✓)
Crunch	(60)	20	2–3	___
Diagonal Crunch	(67)	20	2–3	___
Hand Crunch	(62)	20	2–3	___
Bicycle	(65)	20	2–3	___

35 Minutes of Aerobic Training   ___

DAY 8

5 Minute Aerobic Warm-Up   ____

Weight Training

Exercise	Demo on pg	Reps	# of Sets	Weight	Stretch on pg	(✓)
Butt Kick	(52)	20 Paces	3		(46)	____
Squat #2	(57)	W:20 M:10	2 3	_____	(56)	____
Lying Leg Curls	(45)	W:20 M:10	2 3	_____	(46)	____
Inner Thigh	(47)	20	3	_____	(47)	____
Walking Lunges	(39)	30 Paces	2		(40)	____
Calf Raise	(50)	20 each leg	3		(50)	____
Seated Row	(73)	W:20 M:10	2 3	_____	(72)	____
Hyper-extension	(77)	W:10 M:20	2 3	_____	(72)	____
Cable Curls	(113)	W:20 M:10	2 3	_____	(110)	____
Hammer Curls	(112)	W:20 M:10	2 3	_____	(110)	____

Abdominal Training

Exercise	Demo on pg	Reps	# of Sets	(✓)
Butt Lifts	(64)	20	2–3	____
Toe Touches	(63)	20	2–3	____
Side Crunch	(68)	20	2–3	____
Roman Chair Sit-ups	(61)	20	2–3	____

35 Minutes of Aerobic Training   ____

HALFWAY POINT

You are now halfway through Phase Two, and you should be seeing and feeling the difference both in the way you look and the way you are feeling after your workout. You should notice a fairly dramatic difference in the way your muscles are beginning to feel. They should definitely be more taut, they should be gaining definition, and if your goal is to create mass, you should be experiencing an increase in the size of the muscles. It is quite possible that those who are close to you may be noticing and commenting on your transformation.

If you began this program at Phase One, you should be experiencing some dramatic changes by this juncture. You have just completed your first month on a nutritional program, and your exercise sessions have incrementally increased in difficulty and duration. It is entirely possible that you have taken off twelve pounds of fat, and many inches. What is even more important is that you have been consistently exercising for at least six weeks. Those who may have been leading a more sedentary life to this point will find that their lives have been forever altered. You may now have energy as opposed to feeling lethargic. You may now feel like taking long sunset walks as opposed to watching television. You may find yourself getting out in the garden, playing with your children, your animals or your friends. You may feel more vital than before. You may find yourself infinitely more motivated. It is quite possible that you have more confidence and are more self-assured. You have taken on an activity that has positively affected many aspects of your life. When you make positive change in your life, it positively affects those around you. The point is to create a chain reaction of positivity.

What you have accomplished is truly a feat worth celebrating, and you should seriously consider rewarding yourself for this achievement. Perhaps a weekend getaway . . . perhaps some new clothes . . . perhaps a challenging outdoor adventure with friends or family.

While you are contemplating how you will reward yourself, think about what has changed in your life over the last six weeks. Think back to the first time you had your measurements taken. Were there any negative thoughts about yourself bouncing around in your head? How is that different today? You are changing your perception of yourself. You are perhaps your harshest critic, and if you can change these negative thoughts about yourself, how will others begin to view you? What you are doing to change your mental outlook is perhaps even more important than the physical transformation you are experiencing. In a seemingly endless procession of small achievements, the workouts you are putting yourself through give

As you are now at the half-way point of Phase Two, take your measurements to objectively gauge your progress.

Weight on the scale   _____
Body fat percentage   _____
Right Bicep   _____   Left Bicep   _____
Right Forearm   _____   Left Forearm   _____
Chest (taken at nipple height)   _____
Chest with Arms (taken just below the clavicle
   at the top of the rib cage)   _____
Waist   _____
Hips   _____
Right Thigh   _____   Left Thigh   _____
Right Calf   _____   Left Calf   _____

Again examine your goals.

Are your goals realistic?

Is your goal attainable? Did you set your goal high enough?

Is your goal still the goal, or would you like to make a new goal?

you a certain amount of momentum to carry you through the rest of your day. I am hopeful that what you have experienced in the gym is becoming more applicable at work and at home. These positive changes did not fall from the sky. You made them happen. With your commitment of time and sweat, you made these changes possible. This is an accomplishment that cannot be taken away. It is time for celebration and rewards. You deserve it.

If you are not seeing the results you are looking for, there could be a number of logical explanations. Are you following the nutritional program to the letter? Are you completing your aerobics? If you are looking for greater muscle tone or greater mass, be patient. In the second half of Phase Two I will be introducing a number of techniques that should get you closer to your goal. You will soon see that I have inserted something called a superset. Simply put, a super-set is when you alternate between two exercises without a break or stretch in between. The superset will always emphasize a certain muscle group in that day's workout.

The two exercises in the superset are listed below the heading. You will perform one set of Exercise #1, one set of Exercise #2, and then stretch as prescribed, until you have performed the prescribed number of sets. This should go a long way toward creating added definition and tone. If you are looking to gain mass, I recommend that you try a technique we call "ladder sets." Ladder sets begin with a heavy but manageable weight for the first set. I suggest performing about 12 repetitions. The second set is done with more weight, performing about 10 repetitions, and the last set is done with the heaviest weight possible, performing as many as 8 repetitions.

If you are not losing fat as rapidly as you would like, I have two suggestions. Let me preface my thoughts by reiterating what has been scientifically proven. If you want to rid yourself of fat, and keep that fat off, you could and should only drop a maximum of two pounds per week. Again, your weight on the scale has little to do with fat loss. You are engaging in a fairly intense resistance program, and you are definitely creating muscle and bone density. Muscle weighs approximately twice what fat weighs, so you may want to take another look at your measurements to reassess your progress. If you are still not satisfied, you may think about increasing the amount of time and/or the number of days devoted to your aerobics. Over the next four weeks, you will see that your prescribed aerobic time will gradually be increased. By the time you finish Phase Two, you should be performing 50 – 60 minutes of continuous aerobic activity at least four days per week. Again, you can safely perform aerobics six days per week. The other area that might be examined is your nutritional program. You can refine your nutritional program almost infinitely. You may want to delve deeper, and be more exacting with your food intake. This is an area that requires experimentation, diligence, persistence, and discipline. The more exacting you can be with your food intake, the greater your result will be. It takes some time to get it right, and it requires patience to measure and monitor your food, but it will be worth the extra effort.

5 Minute Aerobic Warm-Up   ___

Weight Training

Exercise	Demo on pg	Reps	# of Sets	Weight	Stretch on pg	(✔)
SUPERSET						
Lat Pull down	(71)	W:20	2		(72)	___
		M:10	3			
Hyper-extension	(77)	W: 10 – 20	2			___
		M: 10 – 20	3			
One Arm Row	(75)	W:20	2		(72)	
		M:10	3			
Shrugs	(79)	W:20	2		(72)	___
		M:20	2			
Delt Wings	(97)	W:20	2	_____	(95)	___
		M:10	3			
Front Raise	(99)	W:20	2	_____	(95)	___
		M:10	3			
W Shoulders	(94)	W:20	2	_____	(95)	___
		M:10	3			
Concentration Curls	(111)	W:20	2	_____	(110)	___
		M:10	3			
Cable Curls	(113)	W:20	2	_____	(110)	___
		M:10	3			
Curls	(109)	W:20	2	_____	(110)	___
		M:10	3			

Abdominal Training

Exercise	Demo on pg	Reps	# of Sets	(✔)
Crunch	(60)	20	2–3	___
Bicycles	(65)	20	2–3	___
Penguins	(66)	20	2–3	___
Diagonal Crunch	(67)	20	2–3	___

40 Minutes of Aerobic Training   ___

5 Minute Aerobic Warm-Up   ___

Weight Training

Exercise	Demo on pg	Reps	# of Sets	Weight	Stretch on pg	(✓)
Leg Extension	(41)	W:20	2	_____	(40)	___
		M:10	3			
SUPERSET						
Leg Press	(53)	W:20	2	_____	(56)	___
		M:10	3			
Leg Curls	(43)	W:20	2	_____	(46)	___
		M:10	3			
Squat #2	(57)	W:20	2	_____	(56)	___
		M:10	3			
Butt Kicks	(52)	20	3	_____	(56)	___
Inner Thigh	(47)	W:20	3	_____	(47)	___
		M:20	3			
Outer Thigh	(48)	20	3	_____	(48)	___
Pec Deck	(89)	W:20	2	_____	(82)	___
		M:10	3			
Push-ups	(87)	W:10 – 20	3	_____	(82)	___
		M: 10 – 20	3			
C Sweeps	(91)	W:20	2	_____	(82)	___
		M:10	3			
Bench Dips	(104)	W:10 – 20	4	_____	(102)	___
		M: 10 – 20	4			
Tricep Kickback with Twist	(106)	W:20	3	_____	(102)	___
		M:10	4			

Abdominal Training

Exercise	Demo on pg	Reps	# of Sets	(✓)
Hand Crunch	(62)	20	2 – 3	___
Side Crunch	(68)	20	2 – 3	___
Toe Touches	(63)	20	2 – 3	___
Roman Sit-ups	(61)	20	2 – 3	___

40 Minutes of Aerobic Training   ___

5 Minute Aerobic Warm-Up   ___

Weight Training

Exercise	Demo on pg	Reps	# of Sets	Weight	Stretch on pg	(✓)
One-Arm Rows	(75)	W:20	2	_____	(72)	___
		M:10	3			
Hyper-extensions	(77)	W:10 – 20	3	_____	(72)	___
		M: 10 – 20	3			
Seated Row	(73)	W:20	2	_____	(72)	___
		M:10	3			
Shrugs	(79)	W:20	2	_____	(72)	___
		M:20	2			
W Shoulders	(94)	W:20	2	_____	(95)	___
		M:10	3			
SUPERSET						
Lateral Raise	(98)	W:20	2	_____	(95)	___
		M:10	3			
Goal Posts	(96)	W:20	2	_____		___
		M:20	3			
Dumbell Curls	(109)	W:20	2	_____	(110)	___
		M:10	3			
Cable Curls	(113)	W:20	2	_____	(110)	___
		M:10	3			
Concentration Curls	(111)	W:20	2	_____	(110)	___
		M:10	3			

Abdominal Training

Exercise	Demo on pg	Reps	# of Sets	(✓)
Diagonal Crunch	(67)	20	2 – 3	___
Bicycles	(65)	20	2 – 3	___
Butt Lifts	(64)	20	2 – 3	___
Crunches	(60)	20	2 – 3	___

40 Minutes of Aerobic Training   ___

DAY 12

5 Minute Aerobic Warm-Up　　　　　　　　　　　　　　　　　　　____

Weight Training

Exercise	Demo on pg	Reps	# of Sets	Weight	Stretch on pg	(✓)
Incline Fly	(85/86)	W:20	2	_____	(82)	___
		M:10	3			
Flat Bench Press	(81)	W:20	2	_____	(82)	___
		M:10	3			
Decline Fly	(85/86)	W:20	2	_____	(82)	___
		M:10	3			
SUPERSET						
Overhead Tricep Extension	(103)	W:10 – 20	2	_____	(102)	___
		M:10 – 20	3			
Tricep Push-down	(105)	W:20	2	_____		___
		M:10	3			
Tricep Extension	(101)	W:20	2	_____	(102)	___
		M:10	3			
Walking Lunges	(34)	W: 30 steps	2		(40)	___
		M: 30 steps	3			
Squat #3 or #2	(55/57)	W:20	2	_____	(56)	___
		M:10	3			
Leg Curls	(45)	W:20	2	_____	(46)	___
		M:10	3			
Leg Extension	(41)	W:20	2	_____	(40)	___
		M:10	3			
Seated Calf Raise	(51)	W:20	3	_____	(51)	___
		M:20	3			

Abdominal Training

Exercise	Demo on pg	Reps	# of Sets	(✓)
Toe Touches	(63)	20	2 – 3	___
Hand Crunch	(62)	20	2 – 3	___
Roman Chair Sit-ups	(61)	20	2 – 3	___
Side Crunch	(68)	20	2 – 3	___

40 Minutes of Aerobic Training　　　　　　　___

DAY 13

5 Minute Aerobic Warm-Up ___

Weight Training

Exercise	Demo on pg	Reps	# of Sets	Weight	Stretch on pg	(✔)
Lat Pull Downs	(71)	W:20 M:10	2 3	_____	(72)	___
Seated Row	(73)	W:20 M:10	2 3	_____	(72)	___
Hyper-extensions	(77)	W:10 M:20	2 2	_____	(72)	___
Shrugs	(79)	W:20 M:20	3 3	_____	(72)	___
Lateral Raises	(98)	W:20 M:10	2 3	_____	(95)	___
Delt Wings	(97)	W:20 M:10	2 3	_____	(95)	___
Front Raise	(99)	W:20 M:10	2 3	_____	(95)	___
SUPERSET **Curls**	(109)	W:20 M:10	2 3	_____		___
Hammer Curls	(112)	W:20 M:10	2 3	_____	(110)	___
Concentration Curls	(111)	W:20 M:10	2 3	_____	(110)	___

Abdominal Training

Exercise	Demo on pg	Reps	# of Sets	(✔)
Diagonal Crunches	(67)	20	2 – 3	___
Bicycles	(65)	20	2 – 3	___
Butt Lift	(64)	20	2 – 3	___
Crunches	(60)	20	2 – 3	___

40 Minutes of Aerobic Training ___

DAY 14

5 Minute Aerobic Warm-Up ___

Weight Training

Exercise	Demo on pg	Reps	# of Sets	Weight	Stretch on pg	(✓)
Tricep Push-down	(105)	W:20 M:10	2 3	___	(102)	___
Tricep Kickback with Twist	(106)	W:20 M:10	2 3	___	(102)	___
Bench Dips	(104)	W:10 – 20 M:10 – 20	3 3	___	(102)	___
SUPERSET **Pec Deck**	(89)	W:20 M:10	2 3	___	(82)	___
Push-ups	(87)	W:10 – 20 M:10 – 20	2 3	___	(82)	___
Decline Press	(84)	W:20 M:10	2 3	___	(82)	___
Inner Thigh	(47)	W:20 M:20	3 3	___	(47)	___
Outer Thigh	(48)	W:20 M:20	3 3	___	(48)	___
Leg Press	(53)	W:20 M:10	2 3	___	(56)	___
Walking Lunges	(39)	W: 30 paces M: 30 paces	3 3		(40)	___
Standing Calf Raises	(50)	W:20 M:20	2 2		(50)	___

Abdominal Training

Exercise	Demo on pg	Reps	# of Sets	(✓)
Penguins	(66)	20	2 – 3	___
Hand Crunches	(62)	20	2 – 3	___
Toe Touches	(63)	20	2 – 3	___
Roman Chair	(61)	20	2 – 3	___

40 Minutes of Aerobic Training ___

DAY 15

5 Minute Aerobic Warm-Up ⎯⎯

Weight Training

Exercise	Demo on pg	Reps	# of Sets	Weight	Stretch on pg	(✓)
Cable Curls	(113)	W:20	2	_____	(110)	⎯⎯
		M:10	3			
Curls	(109)	W:20	2	_____	(110)	⎯⎯
		M:10	3			
Concentration Curls	(111)	W:20	2	_____	(110)	⎯⎯
		M:10	3			
SUPERSET						
One Arm Row	(75)	W:20	2	_____		⎯⎯
		M:10	3			
Shrugs	(79)	W:20	2	_____	(72)	⎯⎯
		M:20	3			
Lat Pull-Downs	(71)	W:20	2	_____	(72)	⎯⎯
		M:10	3			
Hyper-extensions	(77)	W:10 – 20	3	_____	(72)	⎯⎯
		M:10 – 20	3			
W Shoulders	(94)	W:20	2	_____	(95)	⎯⎯
		M:10	3			
Lat Raise	(98)	W:20	2	_____	(95)	⎯⎯
		M:10	3			
Goal Posts	(96)	W:20	2	_____	(95)	⎯⎯
		M:10	3			

Abdominal Training

Exercise	Demo on pg	Reps	# of Sets	(✓)
Diagonal Crunches	(60)	20	2 – 3	⎯⎯
Side Crunch	(68)	20	2 – 3	⎯⎯
Bicycles	(65)	20	2 – 3	⎯⎯
Penguins	(66)	20	2 – 3	⎯⎯
Toe Touches	(63)	20	2 – 3	⎯⎯

50 Minutes of Aerobic Training ⎯⎯

5 Minute Aerobic Warm-Up   ___

Weight Training

Exercise	Demo on pg	Reps	# of Sets	Weight	Stretch on pg	(✓)
SUPERSET						
Squat #2 or #3	(57/58)	W:20	2	_____	(56)	___
		M:10	3			
Butt Kick	(52)	W:20	2	_____		___
		M:20	3			
Leg Curls	(43)	W:20	2	_____	(46)	___
		M:10	3			
SUPERSET						
Leg Extension	(41)	W:20	2	_____		___
		M:10	3			
Inner Thigh	(47)	W:20	2	_____	(40)	___
		M:20	3			
Seated Calf Raise	(51)	W:20	3		(51)	___
		M:20	3			
Push-ups	(87)	W:10 – 20	2		(82)	___
		M:10 – 20	3			
C Sweep	(91)	W:20	2	_____	(82)	___
		M:10	3			
Incline Press	(83)	W:20	2	_____	(82)	___
		M:10	3			
Tricep Extensions	(101)	W:20	2	_____	(102)	___
		M:10	3			
Overhead Tricep Extension	(103)	W:20	2	_____	(102)	___
		M:10	3			

Abdominal Training

Exercise	Demo on pg	Reps	# of Sets	(✓)
Hyper-extension	(77)	20	2 – 3	___
Roman Chair	(61)	20	2 – 3	___
Butt Lift	(64)	20	2 – 3	___
Diagonal Crunches	(67)	20	2 – 3	___
Crunches	(60)	20	2 – 3	___

60 Minutes of Aerobic Training   ___

FINISH LINE

Congratulations! You have completed Phase Two. This is a time for celebration.

This celebration should also involve some honest reflection. How do you feel today, as opposed to just four short weeks ago? Remember when you took your measurements and considered any negative thoughts that were present in your head? Are you free of those negative thoughts? How do you think you look? How do your clothes fit? What is your energy level like now, as opposed to when you first started the program? Compare your job or scholastic performance to that of four weeks ago. Do words like "desire" and "drive" have a different meaning for you today as opposed to when you first started? How does it feel for you to set and meet a certain set of goals several times a week? Has your image of yourself or the respect you have for yourself changed over the last four weeks?

Take a really close look at these numbers. Can you now see what a little effort can result in? When you first began this program, you had a vision of what you would like your body to look like, and you set some goals. If you have not achieved your ultimate goals, how close did you get? How much progress have you made? You have achieved! The differences you may see in your measurements are significant. It is likely that you have not reached your ultimate goals, but your progress marks significant improvement over where you were just four short weeks ago.

The most important thing you have accomplished, however, is that you have incorporated exercise and a new way of eating into your life, and you have exercised regularly for four or eight weeks. This routine has now become a habit. Habits are addicting, so be forewarned that soon you are going to be craving your workouts, and that urge will only become stronger. Unlike any other addiction, this one is good for you. This addiction creates euphoria, improves your sexual drive, makes you feel fantastic, helps you sleep, and will leave you looking better and better each time you get your fix. What is even more intoxicating, however, is that in just one short hour you will have set and attained many goals. The intoxication of achievement and success, and the momentum this creates, will reverberate throughout and positively affect every aspect of your life. What you are now experiencing is truly a positive addiction.

What Next?

At this point, it is important to determine what you would like to do next, and to determine what level of fitness you would like to attain. You may want to take your workouts to a higher level, and feel that it is time for a new challenge. You may find that your personal time constraints or the goals you have set for yourself can be accommodated by the four-days-per-week workout schedule of Phase Two. Whatever your decision, this program will fully meet your needs.

If you desire a new challenge and want to take your physical transformation to the next level, Phase Three will definitely suit you. As this program is designed to take a sedentary reader to the fitness level of a professional athlete in just 12 weeks, choosing to advance to Phase Three will place you amongst the fittest people in the nation. In Phase Three you will be exercising five days per week, and each session will last approximately fifteen minutes longer than your present sessions.

There are some who are very comfortable working out four days per week and find that their goals and needs are met at this level of exercise. For some, attaining this level of fitness is a minor miracle. It has given them the quality of life and level of fitness they have been yearning for. If you choose to remain in Phase Two, there are several adjustments you will need to make, insuring that you will continue to experience results and avoid reaching a training plateau. By this time, you will have realized that no two workouts you have performed to this point have been the same. The purpose of structuring your workouts this way was to continually surprise your body and to prevent you from working out in the same manner on successive days. I recommend repeating the cycle of workouts in Phase Two. After you repeat the sixteen sessions, begin again, but reverse the order of the exercises for each set. On your next series of sixteen sessions, invert the first and second muscle groups being worked. Over the next four-week period, perform the exercises as written. Then repeat the entire process. By merely switching the order of weight-training exercises, you will continually shock the muscles and never become bored in your workouts.

It is now time for you to see your progress on paper.

AFTER

It is so important to be clear about where you are at this moment of your transformation and to be keenly aware of just how far you have come. Allowing yourself to see what you have accomplished in only four weeks will enable you set new goals for what you would like to accomplish next.

Weight on the scale   _____

Body fat percentage   _____

Right Bicep   _____   Left Bicep   _____

Right Forearm   _____   Left Forearm   _____

Chest (taken at nipple height)   _____

Chest with Arms (taken just below the
    clavicle at the top of the rib cage)   _____

Waist   _____

Hips   _____

Right Thigh   _____   Left Thigh   _____

Right Calf   _____   Left Calf   _____

Now compare the numbers you have just written with the numbers you inserted on the "Before" page four weeks ago.

9

Phase Three—5 day a week workout routines

If you began your transformation starting with Phase One, and are now about to try Phase Three, you are going through what is possibly the greatest change of your life. At no other time can you experience the exponential growth that you are presently enjoying. The amount of weight you are lifting now is probably at least 100% more than when you started. The amount of time you can continuously perform aerobic activity has probably doubled. You have reduced by many clothing sizes, and yet you are much stronger and more fit than you were just a short time ago. If you are advancing to Phase Three, chances are that you have either met and surpassed your goals or you are quickly closing in on your goals. Over the next four weeks, this transformational process will become quite exciting, and you may indeed double the results that you have seen thus far. If you are an athlete or someone who has already been exercising regularly, you are about to take a giant step toward your ultimate goal. For you, attaining your goals means to merely make small adjustments to your training regimen to take you to the next level. As a trainer, the questions that are most interesting for me to ponder are how an athlete can improve their game. How does a world-class runner improve her training to compete in the Olympics? What changes could be made in the training of a champion figure skater so that he can bring home the gold? What changes could a minor-league baseball player make in his training regimen so that he could make it in the majors? What does a bodybuilder do to get ready for a show? How can a swimmer take a full second off her time? How does a boxing champion constantly improve quickness, speed, and agility so that he can retain his title? How does a basketball player improve her vertical leap? I have designed Phase Three to be the foundation, to serve as a springboard to make these incredible leaps.

Phase Three is not for the faint of heart. If Phase One created a habit and Phase Two made you an addict, Phase Three is for hard-core junkies only. Phase Three requires you to increase your workout to five days a week. Each session will consist of at least forty-five minutes of aerobic exercise, at least eight minutes of abdominal training, and approximately one hour of weight training. During these five days, I recommend that you spend three days on, one day off, two days on, and one day off. I have found that exercising Monday through Wednesday, resting on Thursday, continuing Friday and Saturday, and resting on Sunday is the optimal schedule for this phase. During your five-day schedule you will do your aerobics and abdominal work, then train each muscle group at least two times per week as part of your weight training. Because of the time involved and to ease the burden of scheduling, this portion of the program is the least structured and grants the most discretion to work towards your ultimate goal unfettered by regimen. No matter how you decide to structure and schedule your week, you *must* rest the body *at least* one full day. This phase of the Hot Point Program is set up as a basic guideline. Based upon your goals, there are specific directions and instruction provided so that you may maximize your effort in reaching your goals and objectives.

When you begin Phase Three, it is essential that you become very clear about your objectives. You have reached this point through some very hard work and dedication, and you should congratulate yourself. It has been at least eight weeks since you began this program, and you are really feeling and seeing the results of your effort. Think back eight weeks. Remembering how you felt at that time, reflect on how you feel now. How did you feel about yourself then, and how do you feel about yourself now? How motivated were you then, and how willing are you now to face challenges and obstacles? Setting out to do something every day, and experiencing that level of achievement, changes your life. Really reflect on the profundity of these changes and how they have affected the quality of your life. It is now time to check the numbers. After taking your measurements and your body-fat percentage, you will have a clear and tangible idea of just how far you have come. It is quite possible that you have lost at least 16 pounds of body fat, you are immeasurably stronger, and the size and proportion of your muscles have been altered to such an extent that people who have not seen your for two months are having difficulty recognizing you. Rewarding yourself may mean a shopping spree, a vacation, or taking up a new sport or activity that utilizes this newly gained strength and mobility.

After rewarding yourself, it is time to reassess where it is that you want to go. This level of training requires that you be very, very specific in terms of your intention and your goals, and that you clearly state the reason why you are attempting to attain such an advanced level of fitness. Phase Two is an excellent permanent program, and achieving that level puts you in the top percentiles of fitness. In Phase Three, you are achieving the training level that professional athletes adhere to. The level of commitment, endurance, and arduousness requires that your objectives be clearly defined. You may want to just challenge yourself even further. You may have seen changes that you didn't think possible, and now you may really want to take an extra step toward having the ultimate body. You may want to become faster or quicker. You may want to increase the size of the muscles in certain areas of the body. You may want to make the varsity team, or you may want a shot at the pros. Whatever the case may be, it is vital to be clear about your objectives and to focus upon them unwaveringly. Even attempting Phase Three is not like tilting with windmills, chasing the brass ring, or attempting the impossible. There are some people who cannot even ponder regular exercise unless they are striving to attain this level of fitness. Unquestionably, you will be taking your level of fitness and commitment to another level altogether. Throughout this phase, and to achieve your goals, you will need to keep your eyes on the prize.

If you can consistently exercise at this level, you will be in the top half of the top 1% of the people in this country who are the most fit. Being able to exercise at this level does not in any way mean that you have crossed a finish line and that this is the end of your journey. This is the level at which I train semipro and professional ball players in the off-season, so they can dramatically improve their game. This is the level at which they begin, and with a little help and guidance, take their game to heights previously unknown to them. Celebrities also feel most comfortable training at this level. The reason is simple. Both of these professions require bodies to look and perform fantastically in order for them to make a living or demand those astronomical salaries. If you are a performer or athlete, or you just want to look really, really amazing, you may consider adding an extra day of aerobic activity to lean out even further and accentuate your muscular definition. Be assured that if you are exercising at this level you are in peak condition.

Once you attain this level, you will just become so enthralled with the way that you feel and feel about yourself that this will become a way of life. It will be a part of your day that cannot be sacrificed for anything or anyone. You will just not feel the same way if you begin to slip. If I do not work out at least five days per week, I begin to feel groggy and sluggish, and I know that I am just not living up to my potential. Potential is a terrible thing to waste. The clearer you are about your goals, the more obvious the reason for you to continue with your transformation. If you know what you are striving for and are clear about your intentions, you know just how much it would mean to you if you could achieve your goals. You are so close to reaching those goals that you can almost touch them. Over the next four weeks I want you to not only touch those goals but to be embracing them.

Watch Out for Overtraining

The only cautionary advice I will give you as you enter Phase Three is to be certain that you are not over-training. There are a few red flags that you should be aware of that indicate over-training. If you begin to have a lack of sleep, if you always seem to be injuring yourself, if you have a lack of motivation to go to the gym, if you are trying to rush through your workout just to get out of the gym, if you are losing lean muscle mass, if you are not able to lift as much weight as when you were in Phase Two you could be overtraining. Overtraining simply means that your body is not ready for this jump. By no means does this mean that you are a failure. You know how much you desire this level of exercise. Your body is just not ready at this time. Your body just needs time to adjust to the new demands you are placing upon it. I suggest going back to the last two weeks of Phase Two. After these two weeks, try taking on Phase Three again. Sometimes it is just a small hump to get over. In other cases, it is an obstacle. Have no fear, if you truly want to be exercising at Phase Three it is only a matter of time.

Like Phases One and Two, I will take you through each step of the process, exercise by exercise, workout by workout. Before you begin, you need to reaffirm your commitment to meet your goals. Be very clear about them. When you are doing your aerobics, daydream a little bit and see in your mind's eye what your life would look like if you could achieve those goals. Write your goals down and tape them to your bathroom mirror and to your refrigerator. The more you are reminded of what you are working so hard to achieve, the easier it will be to reach those goals.

In Phase Three you will want to be working out five days per week. Try to spend three days in a row at the gym, one day off, two days at the gym back to back, and one day at rest. I find that working out Monday through Wednesday, taking Thursday off, working out Friday and Saturday, and taking Sunday off fits my personal schedule. In Phase Three you will want to spend about one hour performing resistance training, and devote at least 45 minutes to your aerobic training. Some may just not have a block of two solid hours in their schedule, so you may have to do your aerobics at a different time in the day. It is really up to you. The important thing is to schedule it in for the next two weeks and let nothing stop you from honoring your commitment. Consult your calendar, day planner or computerized scheduling device, and make an appointment with yourself to reach your goals. By writing in the dates and times, you will have made a binding contract between you and yourself.

Week One   Week Two

_____   _____

_____   _____

_____   _____

_____   _____

_____   _____

Each person reading this book will have different goals, and I will try to address these. This program will only work if you do the exercises that are prescribed, complete your abdominal workout, fulfill or surpass the amount of time that is suggested for aerobic activity, and stick with the nutritional program. If I were by your side, there would be another dynamic in this relationship. I would make sure that you did every repetition of each exercise. I would watch you com-

(continues)

plete your aerobics. And before we started each workout, I would ask you what you had eaten that day and give you suggestions to improve what you eat. On occasion I would even have dinner with you after your workout. Remember that you are doing this to please yourself, and the only person that you have to answer to is yourself. I don't know about you, but I am my harshest critic and my fiercest competitor. By this time you have learned some significant self-motivation techniques and have an enormous amount of drive. I urge you to go the extra mile. Be conscientious about what you are putting into your body. If you are following the direction for your workout and watching your diet, the suggestions I will make half-way through this chapter will be more meaningful.

Take your measurements at this point, before you begin your first workout in Phase Three. Halfway through, in two weeks, you will take those measurements again. You may then make minor adjustments to further your goals. A third set of measurements will be taken at the end of Phase Three so you can see just how far you've come.

PHASE THREE—1ST MEASUREMENT

It is so important to be clear about where you are at this moment of your transformation. **Allowing yourself to take an honest and objective look at this starting point will not only enable you to set and achieve reasonable goals, but will serve as the most effective method to assess your progress towards those goals.**

Weight on the scale _____

Body fat percentage _____

Right Bicep _____   Left Bicep _____

Right Forearm _____   Left Forearm _____

Chest (taken at nipple height) _____

Chest with Arms (taken just below the clavicle
  at the top of the rib cage) _____

Waist _____

Hips _____

Right Thigh _____   Left Thigh _____

Right Calf _____   Left Calf _____

Note: In the Reps column, M=men, W=women

DAY 1

5 Minute Aerobic Warm-Up   ___

Men

Exercise	Demo on pg	Reps	# of Sets	Weight	Stretch on pg	(✓)
Flat Bench Press	(81)	10	2	_____	(82)	___
Pec Deck	(89)	10	4	_____	(82)	___
Incline Flies	(85/86)	10	4	_____	(82)	___
C Sweep	(91)	10	4	_____	(82)	___
Push-ups	(88)	10 – 20	4	_____	(82)	___
Tricep Extension	(101)	10	4	_____	(102)	___
Tricep Push-downs	(105)	10	4	_____	(102)	___
Bench Dips	(104)	20	4	_____	(102)	___
Tricep Kickback with Twist	(106)	10	4	_____	(106)	___

Women

Exercise	Demo on pg	Reps	# of Sets	Weight	Stretch on pg	(✓)
Pec Deck	(89)	20	3	_____	(82)	___
Incline Dumbell Press	(83)	20	3	_____	(82)	___
Push-ups	(87)	20	3	_____	(82)	___
Flat Flies	(85)	20	3	_____	(82)	___
Overhead Tricep Extension	(103)	20	3	_____	(102)	___
Tricep Push-downs	(105)	20	3	_____	(102)	___
Bench Dips	(104)	20	3	_____	(102)	___
Tricep Extension	(101)	20	3	_____	(102)	___

Abdominal Training

Exercise	Demo on pg	Reps	# of Sets	(✓)
Crunches	(60)	20	3 – 4	___
Bicycles	(65)	20	3 – 4	___
Side Crunches	(68)	20	3 – 4	___
Roman Chair	(61)	20	3 – 4	___

45 Minutes of Aerobic Training   ___

5 Minute Aerobic Warm-Up ⎯⎯

Men

Exercise	Demo on pg	Reps	# of Sets	Weight	Stretch on pg	(✔)
Leg Extension	(41)	10	4	_____	(40)	___
Squats #3	(58)	10 – 12	4	_____	(56)	___
Leg Curls	(43)	10	4	_____	(46)	___
Walking Lunges with Weights	(39)	30 steps	4	_____	(40)	___
Outer Thigh	(48)	20	4	_____	(48)	___
Calf Raises	(50)	20	4	_____	(50)	___
W Shoulders	(94)	10	4	_____	(95)	___
Lateral Raises	(98)	10	4	_____	(95)	___
Delt Wings	(97)	10	4	_____	(95)	___
Front Raise	(99)	10 – 12	4	_____	(95)	___

Women

Exercise	Demo on pg	Reps	# of Sets	Weight	Stretch on pg	(✔)
Inner Thigh	(47)	20	4	_____	(47)	___
Outer Thigh	(48)	20	4	_____	(48)	___
Walking Lunge	(39)	15 each leg	3	_____	(40)	___
SUPERSET						
Leg Curl	(43)	20	3	_____	(46)	___
Squat #2	(57)	20	3	_____	(56)	___
Leg Extension	(41)	20	3	_____	(40)	___
Standing Calf Raises	(50)	20	3	_____	(50)	___
Lateral Raises	(98)	20	3	_____	(95)	___
W Shoulders	(94)	20	3	_____	(95)	___
Goal Posts	(96)	20	3	_____	(95)	___

Abdominal Training

Exercise	Demo on pg	Reps	# of Sets	(✔)
Roman Chair	(61)	20	3 – 4	___
Diagonal Crunch	(67)	20	3 – 4	___
Hand Crunch	(62)	20	3 – 4	___
Penguins	(66)	20	3 – 4	___

45 Minutes of Aerobic Training ___

DAY 3

5 Minute Aerobic Warm-Up   ———

Men

Exercise	Demo on pg	Reps	# of Sets	Weight	Stretch on pg	(✓)
SUPERSET						
Seated Rows	(73)	10 – 12	4	_____		———
Hyper-extensions	(77)	20	4	_____	(72)	———
One Arm Rows	(75)	10	4	_____	(72)	———
Lat Pull Down	(71)	10 – 12	4	_____	(72)	———
Shrugs	(79)	20	4	_____		———
Curls	(109)	10	4	_____	(110)	———
Concentration Curls	(111)	10	4	_____	(110)	———
Cable Curl	(113)	10	4	_____	(110)	———
Cable Forearm	(115)	20	4	_____	(115)	———

Women

Exercise	Demo on pg	Reps	# of Sets	Weight	Stretch on pg	(✓)
Lat Pull Down	(71)	20	3 – 4	_____	(72)	———
Seated Rows	(73)	20	3 – 4	_____	(72)	———
One-Arm Row	(75)	20	3 – 4	_____	(72)	———
Hyper-extension	(77)	10 – 20	3 – 4	_____	(72)	———
Cable Curls	(113)	20	3 – 4	_____	(110)	———
Hammer Curls	(112)	20	3	_____	(110)	———
Curls	(109)	20	3	_____	(110)	———
Cable Forearm (optional)	(115)	20	3	_____	(115)	———

Abdominal Training

Exercise	Demo on pg	Reps	# of Sets	(✓)
Side Crunches	(68)	20	3 – 4	———
Butt Lifts	(64)	20	3 – 4	———
Bicycles	(65)	20	3 – 4	———
Crunches	(60)	20	3 – 4	———

45 Minutes of Aerobic Training   ———

DAY 4

5 Minute Aerobic Warm-Up ___

Men

Exercise	Demo on pg	Reps	# of Sets	Weight	Stretch on pg	(✓)
Incline Press	(83)	10	4	_____	(82)	___
Decline Fly	(85/86)	10	4	_____	(82)	___
Flat Bench Press	(81)	10	4	_____	(82)	___
Bench Dips	(104)	10 – 20	4	_____	(102)	___
Tricep Push-downs	(105)	10	4	_____	(102)	___
Tricep Extension	(101)	10	4	_____	(102)	___
SUPERSET						
Leg Press	(53)	10	4	_____	(56)	___
Seated Calf						
Raises	(51)	20	4	_____	(51)	___
Walking Lunges	(39)	30	4	_____	(40)	___
Leg Curls	(43)	10	4	_____	(46)	___

Women

Exercise	Demo on pg	Reps	# of Sets	Weight	Stretch on pg	(✓)
Pec Deck	(89)	20	3 – 4	_____	(82)	___
Flat Bench Press	(81)	20	3 – 4	_____	(82)	___
C Sweeps	(91)	20	3	_____	(82)	___
Tricep Extension	(101)	20	3	_____	(102)	___
Kickback						
with Twist	(106)	20	3	_____	(102)	___
Tricep Push-downs	(105)	20	3	_____	(102)	___
SUPERSET						
Butt Kicks	(52)	20	3	_____		___
Squats #2	(57)	20	3	_____	(56)	___
Inner Thigh	(47)	20	3	_____	(47)	___
Outer Thigh	(48)	20	3	_____	(48)	___
Leg Curls	(43)	20	3	_____	(46)	___
Standing Calf	(50)	20	3	_____	(50)	___

Abdominal Training

Exercise	Demo on pg	Reps	# of Sets	(✓)
Penguins	(66)	20	3 – 4	___
Toe Touches	(63)	20	3 – 4	___
Diagonal Crunches	(67)	20	3 – 4	___
Roman Chair	(61)	20	3 – 4	___

45 Minutes of Aerobic Training ___

5 Minute Aerobic Warm-Up ___

Men

Exercise	Demo on pg	Reps	# of Sets	Weight	Stretch on pg	(✓)
Lat Pull-downs	(71)	10	4	_____	(72)	___
One-Arm Rows	(75)	10	4	_____	(72)	___
Hyper-extensions	(77)	20	4	_____	(72)	___
SUPERSET						
W Shoulders	(94)	10	4	_____		___
Delt Wings	(97)	10	4	_____	(95)	___
Lateral Raises	(98)	10	4	_____	(95)	___
Front Raises	(99	10	4	_____	(95)	___
Cable Curls	(113)	10	4	_____	(110)	___
Concentration Curls	(111)	10	4	_____	(110)	___
Hammer Curls	(112)	10	4	_____	(110)	___
Forearm Cable Curls	(115)	20	4	_____	(115)	___

Women

Exercise	Demo on pg	Reps	# of Sets	Weight	Stretch on pg	(✓)
Seated Row	(73)	20	3	_____	(72)	___
Lat Pull Downs	(71)	20	3	_____	(72)	___
Hyper-extension	(77)	20	3	_____	(72)	___
Goal Posts	(96)	20	3	_____	(95)	___
W Shoulders	(94)	20	3	_____	(95)	___
Front Raises	(99)	20	3	_____	(95)	___
Concentration Curls	(111)	20	3	_____	(110)	___
Hammer Curls	(112)	20	3	_____	(110)	___
(forearms optional)	(115)					

Abdominal Training

Exercise	Demo on pg	Reps	# of Sets	(✓)
Penguin	(62)	20	3 – 4	___
Crunch	(60)	20	3 – 4	___
Bicycles	(65)	20	3 – 4	___
Side Crunch	(68)	20	3 – 4	___

45 Minutes of Aerobic Training ___

DAY 6

5 Minute Aerobic Warm-Up _____

Men

Exercise	Demo on pg	Reps	# of Sets	Weight	Stretch on pg	(✓)
Pec Deck	(89)	10	4	_____	(82)	___
Incline Press	(83)	10	4	_____	(82)	___
Flat Fly	(85)	10	4	_____	(82)	___
SUPERSET						
C Sweep	(91)	10	4	_____		___
Push-ups	(88)	10 – 20	4	_____	(82)	___
Tricep Push-down	(105)	10	4	_____	(102)	___
Tricep Kickbacks						
with Twist	(106)	10	4	_____	(102)	___
Tricep Extensions	(101)	10	4	_____	(102)	___
Overhead Tricep						
Extension	(103)	10	4	_____	(102)	___

Women

Exercise	Demo on pg	Reps	# of Sets	Weight	Stretch on pg	(✓)
Decline Fly	(85/86)	20	3	_____	(82)	___
Push-ups	(87)	10 – 20	3	_____	(82)	___
Incline Press	(83)	20	3	_____	(82)	___
Flat Fly	(85)	20	3	_____	(82)	___
Bench Dips	(104)	20	3	_____	(102)	___
Overhead Tricep						
Extension	(103)	20	3	_____	(102)	___
Tricep Kickbacks						
with Twist	(106)	20	3	_____	(102)	___
Tricep Push-downs	(105)	20	3	_____	(102)	___

Abdominal Training

Exercise	Demo on pg	Reps	# of Sets	(✓)
Hyper-extensions	(77)	20	3 – 4	___
Roman Chair	(61)	20	3 – 4	___
Penguins	(66)	20	3 – 4	___
Diagonal Crunches	(67)	20	3 – 4	___
Toe Touches	(63)	20	3 – 4	___

45 Minutes of Aerobic Training _____

5 Minute Aerobic Warm-Up   ___

Men

Exercise	Demo on pg	Reps	# of Sets	Weight	Stretch on pg	(✓)
Leg Press	(53)	10	4	_____	(56)	___
Leg Extension	(41)	10	4	_____	(40)	___
Leg Curls	(43)	10	4	_____	(46)	___
Inner Thigh	(47)	20	3	_____	(47)	___
Outer Thigh	(48)	20	3	_____	(48)	___
Walking Lunges	(39)	15	3	_____	(40)	___
Calf Raises	(50)	20	4	_____	(50)	___
SUPERSET						
Front Raises	(99)	10	4	_____		___
Delt Wings	(97)	10	4	_____	(95)	___
W Shoulders	(94)	10	4	_____	(95)	___
Goal Posts	(96)	20	4	_____	(95)	___

Women

Exercise	Demo on pg	Reps	# of Sets	Weight	Stretch on pg	(✓)
Walking Lunges	(39)	30	4	_____	(40)	___
SUPERSET						
Outer Thigh	(48)	20	3	_____	(48)	___
Inner Thigh	(47)	20	3	_____	(47)	___
Squats #2	(57)	20	3	_____	(56)	___
Leg Extensions	(41)	20	3	_____	(40)	___
Leg Curls	(43)	20	3	_____	(46)	___
Seated Calf Raises	(51)	20	3	_____	(51)	___
W Shoulders	(94)	20	3	_____	(95)	___
Delt Wings	(97)	20	3	_____	(95)	___
Lateral Raises	(98)	20	3	_____	(95)	___

Abdominal Training

Exercise	Demo on pg	Reps	# of Sets	(✓)
Butt Lifts	(64)	20	3 – 4	___
Bicycles	(65)	20	3 – 4	___
Hand Crunch	(62)	20	3 – 4	___
Hyper-extension	(77)	10 – 20	3 – 4	___

45 Minutes of Aerobic Training   ___

DAY 8

5 Minute Aerobic Warm-Up   ___

Men

Exercise	Demo on pg	Reps	# of Sets	Weight	Stretch on pg	(✓)
Hyper-extension	(77)	10 – 20	3 – 4	_____	(72)	___
Lat Pull Down	(71)	10	4	_____	(72)	___
One-Arm Rows	(75)	10	4	_____	(72)	___
Seated Rows	(73)	10	4	_____	(72)	___
Shrugs	(79)	20	4	_____	(72)	___
Curls	(109)	10	4	_____	(110)	___
Hammer Curls	(112)	10	4	_____	(110)	___
Concentration Curl	(111)	10	4	_____	(110)	___
Cable Curls	(113)	10	4	_____	(110)	___
Cable Forearms	(115)	20	3	_____	(115)	___

Women

Exercise	Demo on pg	Reps	# of Sets	Weight	Stretch on pg	(✓)
Lat Pull Downs	(71)	20	3	_____	(72)	___
One-Arm Rows	(75)	20	3	_____	(72)	___
Seated Rows	(73)	20	3	_____	(72)	___
Shrugs	(79)	20	3	_____	(72)	___
Hyper-extension	(77)	10 – 20	3	_____	(72)	___
Concentration Curls	(111)	20	3	_____	(110)	___
Cable Curls	(113)	20	3	_____	(110)	___
Hammer Curls	(112)	20	3	_____	(110)	___
Curls	(109)	20	3	_____	(110)	___

(cable forearms optional)

Abdominal Training

Exercise	Demo on pg	Reps	# of Sets	(✓)
Crunches	(60)	20	3 – 4	___
Side Crunches	(68)	20	3 – 4	___
Hand Crunch	(62)	20	3 – 4	___
Penguins	(66)	20	3 – 4	___

45 Minutes of Aerobic Training   ___

DAY 9

5 Minute Aerobic Warm-Up   ___

Men

Exercise	Demo on pg	Reps	# of Sets	Weight	Stretch on pg	(✓)
Push-ups	(88)	10 – 20	4	_____	(82)	___
Decline Press	(84)	10	4	_____	(82)	___
Incline Fly	(85/86)	10	4	_____	(82)	___
Pec Deck	(89)	10	4	_____	(82)	___
SUPERSET						
Lateral Raises	(98)	10	4	_____		___
W Shoulders	(94)	10	4	_____	(95)	___
Goal Posts	(96)	20	4	_____	(95)	___
Bench Dips	(104)	20	4	_____	(102)	___
Tricep Push-downs	(105)	10	4	_____	(102)	___
Tricep Kickbacks with Twist	(106)	10	4	_____	(102)	___

Women

Exercise	Demo on pg	Reps	# of Sets	Weight	Stretch on pg	(✓)
Pec Deck	(89)	20	3	_____	(82)	___
Flat Bench Pres	(81)	20	3	_____	(82)	___
C Sweep	(91)	20	3	_____	(82)	___
SUPERSET						
Lateral Raises	(98)	20	3	_____		___
Goal Posts	(96)	20	3	_____	(95)	___
Front Raises	(99)	20	3	_____	(95)	___
Tricep Push-downs	(105)	20	3	_____	(102)	___
Tricep Extensions	(101)	20	3	_____	(102)	___
Bench Dips	(104)	20	3	_____	(102)	___

Abdominal Training

Exercise	Demo on pg	Reps	# of Sets	(✓)
Hyper-extension	(77)	20	3 – 4	___
Roman Chair	(61)	20	3 – 4	___
Crunches	(60)	20	3 – 4	___
Toe Touches	(63)	20	3 – 4	___
Butt Lift	(64)	20	3 – 4	___

45 Minutes of Aerobic Training   ___

5 Minute Aerobic Warm-Up ___

Men

Exercise	Demo on pg	Reps	# of Sets	Weight	Stretch on pg	(✓)
Leg Extensions	(41)	20	3	_____	(40)	___
Walking Lunges	(39)	30 steps	4	_____	(40)	___
Outer Thigh	(48)	20	3	_____	(48)	___
Inner Thigh	(47)	20	3	_____	(47)	___
SUPERSET						
Leg Curls	(43)	10	4	_____	(46)	___
Standing Calf	(50)	20	4	_____	(50)	___
One-Arm Rows	(75)	10	4	_____	(72)	___
Seated Row	(73)	10	4	_____	(72)	___
Shrugs	(79)	20	4	_____	(72)	___
Concentration Curls	(111)	10	4	_____	(110)	___
Cable Curls	(113)	10	4	_____	(110)	___
Forearm Cable Curls	(115)	20	4	_____	(115)	___

Women

Exercise	Demo on pg	Reps	# of Sets	Weight	Stretch on pg	(✓)
Butt Kicks	(52)	20	3	_____	(56)	___
Squats #2	(57)	20	3	_____	(56)	___
Inner Thigh	(47)	20	3	_____	(47)	___
Leg Curls	(43)	20	3	_____	(46)	___
Walking Lunges	(39)	30	3	_____	(40)	___
Seated Calf Raise	(50)	20	3	_____	(50)	___
Seated Rows	(73)	20	3	_____	(72)	___
Lat Pull Downs	(71)	20	3	_____	(72)	___
Shrugs	(79)	20	2	_____	(72)	___
Curls	(109)	20	3	_____	(110)	___
Hammer Curls	(112)	20	3	_____	(110)	___
Cable Curls	(113)	20	3	_____	(110)	___

Abdominal Training

Exercise	Demo on pg	Reps	# of Sets	(✓)
Hyper-extension	(77)	10 – 20	3 – 4	___
Penguins	(66)	20	3 – 4	___
Side Crunches	(68)	20	3 – 4	___
Hand Crunches	(62)	20	3 – 4	___

45 Minutes of Aerobic Training ___

HALFWAY POINT

You are now halfway through Phase Three of the program, and you should be seeing and feeling the difference both in the way you look and the way you are feeling after your workout. You should notice a fairly dramatic difference in the way your muscles are beginning to feel. They should definitely be more taut, they should be gaining definition, and if your goal is to create mass you should be experiencing an increase in the size of the muscles. It is quite possible that those who are close to you may be noticing those very same differences.

If you began this program at Phase One, you should either have surpassed your goals or be so close to them that you can taste them. It is entirely possible that you have taken off at least twelve pounds of fat, and quite a few inches. What is even more important is that you have been consistently exercising for at least ten straight weeks. Over this period of time you have consistently increased your resistance and aerobic levels to such an extent that you are among the fittest in the nation. For those who may have lead a more sedentary life to this point, you have completely changed your life. What you have accomplished is truly a feat worth celebrating, and you should seriously consider rewarding yourself for this achievement. Perhaps you should be collecting catalogs and selecting a new wardrobe . . . a vacation where you can flaunt your new body on the beach? While you are contemplating how you will reward yourself, think about what has changed in your life over the last ten weeks.

Think back to the first time you had your measurements taken. Were there any negative thoughts about yourself bouncing around in your head? How is that different today? You are changing your perception of yourself. You are perhaps your harshest critic, and if you can change these negative thoughts about yourself, how will others begin to view you? What you are doing to change your mental outlook is perhaps even more important that the physical transformation you are experiencing. In a seemingly endless procession of small achievements, the workouts you are putting yourself through give you a certain amount of momentum to carry you through the rest of your day. I am hopeful that what you have experienced in the gym is becoming more applicable at work and at home. These positive changes did not fall from the sky. You made them happen. With your commitment of time and sweat, you made these changes possible. This is an accomplishment that cannot be taken away. It is time for celebration and rewards. You deserve it.

Most probably you are on your way to achieving your goal. However, if you are not seeing the results you are looking for, there could be a number of logical explanations. If you are looking for greater muscle tone or greater mass, you will want to make slight adjustments to your prescribed workout. The first suggestion is to incorporate something called pyramid training. For each exercise, begin the set with a weight that is fairly easy to move. Increase the weight for your second set. Increase the weight again for your third set, and perform eight repetitions. On your fourth set, do the weight and reps of the second set. Add a fifth set, and drop the weight so you can perform 15 – 20 repetitions. Another suggestion is to work with heavy weight and perform at least five sets. Your first set is designed to warm up the muscle you are about to work. For this first set use a lighter weight and perform ten repititions. Increase the weight considerably, and perform 6 – 8 repetitions for the next four sets.

If you are not ridding yourself of fat as rapidly as you would like, I have two suggestions. Let me preface my thoughts by reiterating what has been scientifically proven. If you want to rid yourself of fat, and keep that fat off, you could and should only drop a maximum of two pounds per week. Again, your weight on the scale has little to do with fat loss. You are engaging in a fairly intense resistance program, and you are definitely creating muscle and bone density. Muscle weighs approximately twice what fat weighs, so you may want to take another look at your measurements to reassess your progress. If you are still not satisfied, you may think about increasing the amount of time and/or the number of days devoted to your aerobics. I have suggested that you perform at least 45 minutes of aerobic training. If you are looking to bring in your abdominal muscles, you may want to increase your aerobics by about 5 – 10 minutes per day, until you are exercising for a solid hour and fifteen minutes. Perhaps you would like to add an extra aerobic session on one of your "off" days. Perhaps you would like to increase the number of aerobic sessions to two per workout day. Again, you can safely perform aerobics six days per week, but your body will need one day of rest to rejuvenate itself. You also may want to reexamine your nutritional program. You can refine your nutritional program almost infinitely. If you are practicing the simpler 1:1 or 1:2 model, you may want to delve deeper into your own nutritional needs and be more exacting with your food intake. This is an area that requires experimentation, diligence, persistence, and discipline. The more exacting you can be with your food intake, the greater the result. It takes some time to get it right and patience to measure and monitor your food, but it may be worth the extra effort. If you are already using total caloric intake as the basis for your nutritional program, there are a number of adjustments that you can make. The first suggestion I would make is that you reduce the number of calories by 100 and increase your aerobic level 15 minutes per day. Try this for a week and see what the results are. Be certain not to take your caloric intake under 1000 calories per day. If you are not seeing results after two weeks, drop your total caloric intake another 100 calories and increase your aerobic activity another 10 minutes, but do not exceed one hour and fiftenn minutes. Once you begin the process of radically adjusting your calories, or from where you derive your calories, you invite questionable and sometimes harmful nutritional practices. Another method to adjust the total calories is to increase the amount of calories derived from protein by as much as 10%, and decrease the amount of calories derived from carbohydrates by the same amount. The only proviso to this method is not to exceed 50 grams of protein per meal. If such an increase would put you over 50 grams, add another meal. Such experimentation should not be taken lightly, and you should only turn to these options as a last resort.

With these minor adjustments made, it is now time to finish up the last two weeks of Phase Three.

This celebration should also involve some honest reflection. How do you feel today, as opposed to just twelve short weeks ago? Remember when you first took your measurements and considered any negative thoughts that were present in your head? Are you free of those negative thoughts? How do you think you look? How do friends and loved ones say that you look? How do your clothes fit? What is your energy level like now, as opposed to when you first started the program? Compare your job or scholastic performance to that of twelve weeks ago. Do words like "desire" and "drive" have a different meaning for you today as opposed to when you first started? How does it feel for you to have met your goals? Has your image of yourself or the respect you have for yourself changed over the last twelve weeks?

Take a really close look at these numbers. Can you now see what a little effort can result in? When you first began this program, you had a vision of what you would like your body to look like and you set some goals. If you have not achieved your ultimate goals, how close did you get? How much progress have you made? You have achieved! The differences you may see in your measurements are significant. It is likely that you have reached your ultimate goals, and if not, you have gotten very, very close. In either case, your progress marks significant improvement over where you were just a short time ago.

The most important thing you have accomplished, however, is that you have made exercise and proper nutrition a part of your life. Because you have exercised regularly for many weeks, this routine has flourished from a habit to an overwhelming addiction. It is now something that you cannot do without. Unlike any other addiction known to man, this is the only one that is actually good for you. This addiction creates euphoria, improves your sexual drive, makes you feel fantastic, helps you sleep, and will leave you looking better and better each time you get your fix. What is even more intoxicating, however, is the way it makes you feel about yourself and, consequently, how others have begun to feel about you. The intoxication of achievement and success, and the momentum this creates, have reverberated throughout your life and positively affected every aspect of it. You are now a Hot Point Junkie.

What Next?

At this point, it is important to determine where you are and what you would like to do next. Once you have completed Phase Three, you are enjoying a level of fitness that very few people enjoy. It is entirely possible that you have achieved your goals, and if you have, do not be too concerned with maintaining this rigorous workout schedule. Life happens. You may not have enough time to continue working out at this level. Do not fear. By simply reverting back to Phase Two, or a four-day-per-week schedule, you can easily maintain everything you have achieved. When you are ready, willing, and able, and driven to experience a new plateau, begin Phase Three again. You will be blown away by your gains.

If you do choose to remain in Phase Three, there are several adjustments you will need to make to insure that you will continue to experience results and avoid reaching a training plateau. By this time you will have realized that no two workouts you have performed to this point have been the same. The reason your workouts have been structured in this way was to continually surprise your body and to prevent you from working out in the same manner on successive days. I recommend repeating the cycle of workouts in Phase Three. After you repeat the twenty sessions, begin again, but reverse the order of the exercises. On your next series of twenty sessions, invert the first and second muscle groups being worked. Over the next four-week period, perform the exercises as written. Then repeat the entire process. By merely switching the order of weight-training exercises, you will continually shock the muscles and never become bored in your workouts.

As you are now at the half-way point of Phase Three, I recommend that you take your measurements to objectively gauge your progress.

PHASE THREE—2ND MEASUREMENT

Weight on the scale _____

Body fat percentage _____

Right Bicep _____   Left Bicep _____

Right Forearm _____   Left Forearm _____

Chest (taken at nipple height) _____

Chest with Arms (taken just below the clavicle
   at the top of the rib cage) _____

Waist _____

Hips   _____

Right Thigh _____   Left Thigh _____

Right Calf _____   Left Calf _____

DAY 11

5 Minute Aerobic Warm-Up ___

Men

Exercise	Demo on pg	Reps	# of Sets	Weight	Stretch on pg	(✓)
Push-up	(88)	10	3	_____	(82)	___
Incline Press	(83)	10	4	_____	(82)	___
Flat Flies	(85)	10	4	_____	(82)	___
C Sweep	(91)	10	4	_____	(82)	___
W Shoulders	(94)	10	4	_____	(95)	___
Lateral Raises	(98)	10	4	_____	(95)	___
Delt Wings	(97)	10	4	_____	(95)	___
Tricep Push-downs	(105)	10	4	_____	(102)	___
Tricep Extension	(101)	10	4	_____	(102)	___
Overhead Tricep Extension	(103)	10	4	_____	(102)	___

Women

Exercise	Demo on pg	Reps	# of Sets	Weight	Stretch on pg	(✓)
Push-up #1 or #2	(87/88)	20	3	_____	(82)	___
C Sweep	(91)	20	3	_____	(82)	___
Incline Press	(83)	20	3	_____	(82)	___
Bench Dips	(104)	20	3	_____	(102)	___
Overhead Tricep Extension	(103)	20	3	_____	(102)	___
Tricep Extension	(101)	20	3	_____	(102)	___
Delt Wings	(97)	20	3	_____	(95)	___
Lateral Raises	(98)	20	3	_____	(95)	___
Front Raises	(99)	20	3	_____	(95)	___

Abdominal Training

Exercise	Demo on pg	Reps	# of Sets	(✓)
SUPERSET				
Crunches	(60)	60	3 – 4	___
Toe Touches	(63)	20	3 – 4	___
Bicycle	(65)	20	3 – 4	___
Butt Lifts	(64)	20	3 – 4	___

45 Minutes of Aerobic Training ___

5 Minute Aerobic Warm-Up

Men

Exercise	Demo on pg	Reps	# of Sets	Weight	Stretch on pg	(✓)
Seated Row	(73)	10	3	_____	(72)	___
Lat Pull Down	(71)	10	4	_____	(72)	___
Hyper-extension	(77)	10 – 20	4	_____	(72)	___
Shrugs	(79)	20	4	_____	(72)	___
Curls	(104)	10	4	_____	(102)	___
Cable Curls	(113)	10	4	_____	(102)	___
Concentration Curls	(111)	10	4	_____	(102)	___
SUPERSET						
Leg Extensions	(41)	10	4	_____	(40)	___
Leg Press	(53)	10	4	_____	(56)	___
Leg Curls	(43)	10	4	_____	(46)	___
Squat #3	(58)	30	4	_____	(56)	___
Standing Calf Raise	(50)	20	4	_____	(50)	___

Women

Exercise	Demo on pg	Reps	# of Sets	Weight	Stretch on pg	(✓)
One-Arm Rows	(75)	20	3	_____	(72)	___
Lat Pull Downs	(71)	20	3	_____	(72)	___
Hyper-extension	(77)	10 – 20	3	_____	(72)	___
Concentration Curls	(111)	20	3	_____	(110)	___
Curls	(109)	20	3	_____	(110)	___
Hammer Curls	(112)	20	3	_____	(110)	___
Leg Curl	(43)	20	3	_____	(46)	___
Outer Thigh	(48)	20	3	_____	(48)	___
Inner Thigh	(47)	20	3	_____	(47)	___
SUPERSET						
Leg Press	(53)	20	3	_____	(56)	___
Walking Lunges	(39)	30 paces	3	_____	(40)	___
Standing Calf Raises	(50)	20	3	_____	(50)	___

Abdominal Training

Exercise	Demo on pg	Reps	# of Sets	(✓)
Roman Chair Side	(69)	20	3 – 4	___
Crunch	(60)			
Roman Chair Sit-ups	(61)	20	3 – 4	___
Penguins	(66)	20	3 – 4	___
Diagonal Crunch	(67)	20	3 – 4	___

45 Minutes of Aerobic Training   ___

5 Minute Aerobic Warm-Up   ___

Men

Exercise	Demo on pg	Reps	# of Sets	Weight	Stretch on pg	(✓)
SUPERSET						
Shrugs	(79)	20	4	_____		___
W Shoulders	(94)	10	4	_____	(95)	___
Push-ups	(98)	10	3	_____	(95)	___
Goal Post	(96)	20	4	_____	(95)	___
Front Raises	(99)	20	4	_____	(95)	___
Tricep Extension	(101)	10	4	_____	(102)	___
Tricep Push-downs	(105)	10	4	_____	(102)	___
Bench Dips	(104)	20	4	_____	(102)	___
Tricep Kickbacks with Twist	(106)	10	4	_____	(102)	___

Women

Exercise	Demo on pg	Reps	# of Sets	Weight	Stretch on pg	(✓)
SUPERSET						
Shrugs	(79)	20	4	_____		___
Lat Raise	(98)	20	3	_____	(95)	___
W Shoulders	(94)	20	3	_____	(95)	___
Goal Post	(96)	20	3	_____	(95)	___
Front Raise	(99)	20	3	_____	(95)	___
Tricep Kickbacks with Twist	(106)	20	3	_____	(102)	___
Tricep Push-downs	(105)	20	3	_____	(102)	___
Overhead Tricep Extension	(103)	20	3	_____	(102)	___
Bench Dips	(104)	20	3	_____	(102)	___

Abdominal Training

Exercise	Demo on pg	Reps	# of Sets	(✓)
Bicycle	(65)	20	3 – 4	___
Crunch	(60)	20	3 – 4	___
Side Crunch	(68)	20	3 – 4	___
Toe Touches	(63)	20	3 – 4	___

45 Minutes of Aerobic Training   ___

DAY 14

5 Minute Aerobic Warm-Up ____

Men

Exercise	Demo on pg	Reps	# of Sets	Weight	Stretch on pg	(✓)
Flat Bench Press	(81)	10	4	_____	(82)	___
Pec Deck	(89)	10	4	_____	(82)	___
Decline Press	(84)	10	4	_____	(82)	___
SUPERSET						
Push-ups	(88)	10	4			___
Incline Fly	(85/86)	10	4	_____	(82)	___
Cable Curls	(113)	10	4	_____	(110)	___
SUPERSET						
Curls	(109)	10	4	_____	(110)	___
Hammer Curls	(112)	10	4	_____	(110)	___
Concentration Curls	(111)	10	4	_____	(110)	___
Forearm Cable Curls	(115)		3	_____	(115)	___

Women

Exercise	Demo on pg	Reps	# of Sets	Weight	Stretch on pg	(✓)
SUPERSET						
Push-up	(87)	20	3	_____		___
Pec Deck	(89)	20	3	_____	(82)	___
Flat Bench Press	(81)	20	3	_____	(82)	___
Decline Fly	(85/86)	20	3	_____	(82)	___
C Sweep	(91)	20	3	_____	(82)	___
Curls	(109)	20	3	_____	(110)	___
Concentration Curls	(111)	20	3	_____	(110)	___
SUPERSET						
Hammer Curls	(112)	20	3	_____		___
Cable Curls	(113)	20	3	_____	(110)	___
(forearms optional)	(115)					

Abdominal Training

Exercise	Demo on pg	Reps	# of Sets	(✓)
Roman Chair	(61)	20	3 – 4	___
Diagonal Crunch	(67)	20	3 – 4	___
Penguin	(66)	20	3 – 4	___
Butt Lift	(64)	20	3 – 4	___

45 Minutes of Aerobic Training ___

DAY 15

5 Minute Aerobic Warm-Up   ___

Men

Exercise	Demo on pg	Reps	# of Sets	Weight	Stretch on pg	(✓)
Leg Extension	(41)	10	4	_____	(40)	___
Squat #3	(58)	10	4	_____	(56)	___
Leg Curls	(43)	10	4	_____	(46)	___
Outer Thigh	(48)	20	2	_____	(48)	___
Inner Thigh	(47)	20	2	_____	(47)	___
Walking Lunges	(39)	30 paces	3	_____	(40)	___
Standing Calf Raises	(50)	20	4	_____	(50)	___
Seated Row	(73)	10	4	_____	(72)	___
Lat Pull Down	(71)	10	4	_____	(72)	___
One-Arm Rows	(75)	10	4	_____	(72)	___
Shrugs	(79)	10	4	_____	(72)	___

Women

Exercise	Demo on pg	Reps	# of Sets	Weight	Stretch on pg	(✓)
Leg Extension	(41)	20	3	_____	(40)	___
Leg Curls	(43)	20	3	_____	(46)	___
Squats #2	(57)	20	3	_____	(56)	___
Walking Lunges	(39)	30	3	_____	(40)	___
Butt Kicks	(52)	20	3	_____	(56)	___
Calf Raise	(50)	20	3	_____	(50)	___
Seated Row	(73)	20	3	_____	(72)	___
Lat Pull Down	(71)	20	3	_____	(72)	___
Hyper-extension	(77)	10 – 20	3	_____	(72)	___
Shrugs	(79)	20	3	_____	(72)	___

Abdominal Training

Exercise	Demo on pg	Reps	# of Sets	(✓)
Toe Touches	(63)	20	3 – 4	___
Bicycles	(65)	20	3 – 4	___
Hand crunch	(62)	20	3 – 4	___
Roman Chair	(61)	20	3 – 4	___

45 Minutes of Aerobic Training   ___

*Take one day off before moving on to the Day 16 workout.

DAY 16

5 Minute Aerobic Warm-Up   ___

Men

Exercise	Demo on pg	Reps	# of Sets	Weight	Stretch on pg	(✓)
Leg Extension	(41)	10	4	_____	(40)	___
Squat #3	(58)	10	4	_____	(56)	___
Leg Curls	(43)	10	4	_____	(46)	___
Calf Raises	(50)	20	4	_____	(50)	___
Lat Pull Downs	(71)	10	4	_____	(72)	___
Seated Row	(73)	10	4	_____	(72)	___
Hyper-extension	(77)	10 – 20	4	_____	(72)	___
Cable Curls	(113)	10	4	_____	(110)	___
Curls	(109)	10	4	_____	(110)	___
Concentration Curls	(111)	10	4	_____	(110)	___

Women

Exercise	Demo on pg	Reps	# of Sets	Weight	Stretch on pg	(✓)
SUPERSET						
Outer Thigh	(48)	20	3	_____	(48)	___
Butt Kicks	(52)	20	3	_____	(56)	___
Inner Thigh	(47)	20	3	_____	(47)	___
Leg Curls	(43)	20	3	_____	(46)	___
Hyper-extension	(77)	10 – 20	3	_____	(72)	___
Lat Pull Downs	(71)	20	3	_____	(72)	___
One-Arm Rows	(75)	20	3	_____	(72)	___
Cable Curls	(113)	20	3	_____	(110)	___
Hammer Curls	(112)	20	3	_____	(110)	___
Concentration Curls	(111)	20	3	_____	(110)	___

Abdominal Training

Exercise	Demo on pg	Reps	# of Sets	(✓)
Roman Chair	(61)	20	3 – 4	___
Penguins	(66)	20	3 – 4	___
Roman Side Crunches	(69)	20	3 – 4	___
Butt Lifts	(64)	20	3 – 4	___

45 Minutes of Aerobic Training   ___

DAY 17

5 Minute Aerobic Warm-Up ___

Men

Exercise	Demo on pg	Reps	# of Sets	Weight	Stretch on pg	(✓)
Tricep Push-downs	(105)	10	4	_____	(102)	___
Overhead Tricep						
Extension	(103)	10	4	_____	(102)	___
Bench Dips	(104)	10	4	_____	(102)	___
Incline Press	(83)	10	4	_____	(82)	___
C Sweep	(91)	10	4	_____	(82)	___
Pec Deck	(89)	10	4	_____	(82)	___
SUPERSET						
Delt Wing	(97)	10	4	_____		___
W Shoulders	(94)	10	4	_____	(95)	___
Lateral Raises	(98)	10	4	_____	(95)	___
Hyper-extension	(77)	20	3	_____	(72)	___

Women

Exercise	Demo on pg	Reps	# of Sets	Weight	Stretch on pg	(✓)
Tricep Kickback						
with Twist	(106)	20	3	_____	(102)	___
Tricep Extension	(101)	20	3	_____	(102)	___
Overhead Tricep						
Extension	(103)	20	3	_____	(102)	___
Delt Wings	(97)	20	3	_____	(95)	___
SUPERSET						
Lateral Raises	(98)	20	3	_____		___
Front Raises	(99)	20	3	_____	(95)	___
Flat Flies	(85)	20	3	_____	(82)	___
Incline Bench Press	(83)	20	3	_____	(82)	___
Pec Deck	(89)	20	3	_____	(82)	___

Abdominal Training

Exercise	Demo on pg	Reps	# of Sets	(✓)
SUPERSET				
Toe touches	(63)	20	3 – 4	___
Hand crunches	(62)	20	3 – 4	___
Diagonal Crunch	(67)	20	3 – 4	___
Crunches	(60)	20	3 – 4	___

45 Minutes of Aerobic Training ___

DAY 18

5 Minute Aerobic Warm-Up   ___

Men

Exercise	Demo on pg	Reps	# of Sets	Weight	Stretch on pg	(✓)
Cable Curls	(113)	10	4	_____	(110)	___
Concentration Curls	(111)	10	4	_____	(110)	___
Hammer Curls	(112)	10	4	_____	(110)	___
Curls	(109)	10	4	_____	(110)	___
Lat Pull Down	(71)	10	4	_____	(72)	___
One-Arm Rows	(75)	10	4	_____	(72)	___
Seated Rows	(73)	10	4	_____	(72)	___
Shrugs	(79)	10	4	_____	(72)	___
Forearm Cable Curls	(115)	20	4	_____	(115)	___
Hyper-extension	(77)	20	3	_____		___

Women

Exercise	Demo on pg	Reps	# of Sets	Weight	Stretch on pg	(✓)
Hammer Curls	(112)	20	3	_____	(110)	___
Concentration Curl	(111)	20	3	_____	(110)	___
Curls	(109)	20	3	_____	(110)	___
One-Arm Rows	(75)	20	3	_____	(72)	___
Lat Pull Downs	(71)	20	3	_____	(72)	___
Seated Row	(73)	20	3	_____	(72)	___
Shrugs	(79)	20	3	_____	(72)	___
Hyper-extension	(77)	10 – 20	3	_____	(72)	___

Abdominal Training

Exercise	Demo on pg	Reps	# of Sets	(✓)
Roman Side Crunch	(69)	20	3 – 4	___
Roman Chair	(61)	20	3 – 4	___
Bicycles	(65)	20	3 – 4	___
Butt Lift	(64)	20	3 – 4	___

45 Minutes of Aerobic Training   ___

DAY 19

5 Minute Aerobic Warm-Up　　　　　　　　　　　　　　　　　　—

Men

Exercise	Demo on pg	Reps	# of Sets	Weight	Stretch on pg	(✓)
Outer Thigh	(48)	20	3	_____	(48)	___
Inner Thigh	(47)	20	3	_____	(47)	___
Leg Extension	(41)	10	4	_____	(40)	___
SUPERSET						
Leg Press	(53)	10	4	_____	(56)	___
Seated Calf	(51)	20	4	_____	(51)	___
Walking Lunges	(39)	30 paces	3	_____	(40)	___
Front Raises	(99)	10	4	_____	(95)	___
Goal Posts	(96)	10	4	_____	(95)	___
Lateral Raises	(98)	10	4	_____	(95)	___
W Shoulders	(94)	10	4	_____	(95)	___

Women

Exercise	Demo on pg	Reps	# of Sets	Weight	Stretch on pg	(✓)
Leg Extension	(41)	20	3	_____	(40)	___
Walking Lunges	(39)	30	2	_____	(40)	___
Leg Press	(53)	20	3	_____	(56)	___
Butt Kicks	(52)	20	3	_____	(47)	___
Inner Thigh	(47)	20	3	_____	(48)	___
Outer Thigh	(48)	20	3	_____	(51)	___
Seated Calf	(51)	20	3	_____	(95)	___
Front Raises	(99)	20	3	_____	(95)	___
W Shoulders	(94)	20	3	_____	(95)	___
Goal Posts	(96)	20	3	_____	(95)	___

Abdominal Training

Exercise	Demo on pg	Reps	# of Sets	(✓)
Butt Lift	(64)	20	3 – 4	___
Roman Sit-ups	(61)	20	3 – 4	___
Side Crunches	(68)	20	3 – 4	___
Crunches	(60)	20	3 – 4	___

45 Minutes of Aerobic Training　　　　　　　　　　　—

5 Minute Aerobic Warm-Up ____

Men

Exercise	Demo on pg	Reps	# of Sets	Weight	Stretch on pg	(✓)
SUPERSET						
Pec Deck	(89)	10	4	_____		___
Push-ups	(88)	10 – 20	4	_____	(82)	___
Decline Bench Press	(84)	20	3	_____	(82)	___
Flat Bench Press	(81)	10	4	_____	(82)	___
Incline Fly	(85/86)	10	4	_____	(82)	___
Bench Dips	(104)	10	4	_____	(102)	___
Tricep Push-down	(105)	10	4	_____	(102)	___
Overhead Tricep Extension	(103)	10	4	_____	(102)	___
Tricep Kick Back with Twist	(106)	10	4	_____	(102)	___

Women

Exercise	Demo on pg	Reps	# of Sets	Weight	Stretch on pg	(✓)
Incline Fly	(85/86)	20	3	_____	(82)	___
Flat Bench Press	(81)	20	3	_____	(82)	___
C Sweep	(91)	20	3	_____	(82)	___
Push-ups	(87/88)	20	3	_____	(82)	___
Bench Dips	(104)	20	3	_____	(102)	___
Tricep Extension	(101)	20	3	_____	(102)	___
Overhead Tricep Extension	(103)	20	3	_____	(102)	___
Tricep Kickback with Twist	(106)	20	3	_____	(102)	___

Abdominal Training

Exercise	Demo on pg	Reps	# of Sets	(✓)
Penguins	(66)	20	3 – 4	___
Crunches	(61)	20	3 – 4	___
Toe touches	(63)	20	3 – 4	___
Roman Side Crunch	(69)	20	3 – 4	___

45 Minutes of Aerobic Training ____

FINISH LINE

Congratulations! You have completed Phase Three. This is a time for celebration. *It is now time for you to see your progress on paper.*

AFTER

It is so important to be clear about where you are at this moment of your transformation and to be keenly aware of just how far you have come. Allowing yourself to see what you have accomplished in only four weeks will enable you to set new goals for what you would like to accomplish next.

Weight on the scale   _____

Body fat percentage   _____

Right Bicep   _____   Left Bicep   _____

Right Forearm _____   Left Forearm _____

Chest (taken at nipple height)   _____

Chest with Arms (taken just below the clavicle
    at the top of the rib cage)   _____

Waist   _____

Hips   _____

Right Thigh   _____   Left Thigh   _____

Right Calf   _____   Left Calf   _____

Now I would like you to compare the numbers you have just written with the numbers you inserted on the "Before" page when you first started.

10

The Result Zone!

Like a staircase, you have taken many steps, and those steps have led to an amazing destination. You have consciously or unconsciously derived some powerful tools that can and should be applied to every facet of your life. By setting goals and working toward them, by scheduling your time, by experiencing daily victories, and by experiencing some level of physical transformation, something remarkable has happened to you.

What you are experiencing is self-empowerment at its most profound level. It is my belief that we can only control two things in life: our body and our mind. The exercises you have been doing were not only exercises that strengthened your muscles but were exercises that tested and strengthened your will, your desire, and your concentration. Through this control over your mind, you have experienced the control you have over your body and have driven yourself to some level of transformation. If you can control your body, and you can control your mind, you can control your life. When you are in control of your life, you reach another level of living. When you reach that level, you realize that you really don't need anything external to make you happy, you simply realize that you just are actually happy. You are satisfied with your progress, with your effort, and are satisfied with yourself for who and what you are. When you attain this level, you are not merely existing, but *living.* Living life passionately is really the point after all.

When you can live your life passionately, you are able to attain something beyond attaining achievement . . . You are able to take your life to another level. A level that you never knew existed. Analogy to sports is one that translates easily for me. There have been players—the true great ones—who have redefined the sports they were involved with. They did things that people had never seen, and are never likely to see again. They found this level that I speak of. The level which is beyond the level of "very good" or "excellent," they reached a level that transcended the game they played. Think back on the last shot that Michael Jordan ever took. Watch Mark McGuire as he gets into his stance and concentrates on the pitcher. They go to another level and are able to perform the extraordinary. This level of the game is not the exclusive domain of athletes. These great players were not born superstars, but rather developed *into* superstars. The game of life has many players, and all of the players have the chance to become "superstars." This level is not reserved only for the ultra-wealthy, or for powerbrokers. This level is for you.

You have several things in common with the superstar athlete. You have purpose, and have dedicated yourself to achieving a goal. You have been focused and diligent about improving your "game." More impressive than anything else, you have put in the effort and worked very hard. Without these qualities, even the most gifted athlete would never become a star. You have pushed beyond your limits. You have exceeded what you thought you could do. No matter what level you have taken your physical transformation to, you have taken your life to another level. That is truly a success.

The greatest part about being a personal trainer is to form a bond with my clients, to be at their side while they are struggling, to see the improvements they make, and to see firsthand what those changes mean to them and to their lives. I have had the great fortune of seeing many people change their lives through Hot Point Fitness. I encourage you to send your "before" and "after" photographs to the publisher, who just may include them in the next printing. Or, email these photos to atighteru@aol.com. And please be sure to include some thoughts on how this program made a difference in your life.

See you at the gym.